# ADVANCES IN PEDIATRIC SPORT SCIENCES

## VOLUME TWO
## BEHAVIORAL ISSUES

**Daniel Gould, PhD**
University of Illinois at Urbana-Champaign

**Maureen R. Weiss, PhD**
University of Oregon, Eugene
**Editors**

**Human Kinetics Publishers, Inc.**
**Champaign, Illinois**

Developmental Editor: Laura E. Larson
Production Director: Ernie Noa
Assistant Production Director: Lezli Harris
Copy Editor: Laura E. Larson
Typesetter: Brad Colson
Proofreader: Linda Purcell
Text Layout: Denise Mueller
Printed By: Braun-Brumfield, Inc.

Library of Congress Catalog Number: 85-644893
ISBN: 0-87322-089-7
ISSN: 0748-6375
Copyright © 1987 by Human Kinetics Publishers, Inc.

Printed in the United States of America.

10  9  8  7  6  5  4  3  2  1

Human Kinetics Publishers, Inc.
Box 5076, Champaign, IL  61820

# Contents

# About the Series

*Advances in Pediatric Sport Sciences*, or APSS, is an interdisciplinary series published every other year. Scholarly reviews pertaining to children and physical activity will be reported in each volume, with Volume 1 and each subsequent odd-numbered volume focusing on *biological issues* and Volume 2 and each subsequent even-numbered volume focusing on *behavioral issues*.

Topics covered under biological issues include physiological, biomechanical, medical, and some topics within motor control and development as they pertain to pediatric sport sciences. Behavioral issues will draw upon other topics within motor control and development, sport and exercise psychology, sociology of sport, and anthropology of sport and play.

The series is intended to help advance our understanding of children and their health and well-being as they participate in physical activity. Organized sport, play, and fitness activities are common forms of physical activity that will frequently be considered in the series, but they will not be the only forms considered.

The editor for each volume is selected by the publisher. Persons who may be interested in contributing to the series are encouraged to contact the publisher to learn who the editors are for forthcoming volumes.

# Preface

Physical activity is one of the most prevalent and important behaviors observed in children and youth. Every child participates in some type of physical activity, whether it takes the form of informal play, organized sport, exercise or the development of fundamental motor skills. Recognizing the universal importance of physical activity for the child, investigators have begun to examine the cultural, environmental, and personal variables that affect children's participation in and performance of physical activities, as well as how participation in various physical activity forms affects the child's social, psychological, and motor development.

A major finding of the pediatric behavioral science research is that children are not simply miniature adults. As the human organism grows and develops, a variety of cognitive, social-emotional, and physiological changes occurs that directly affect the acquisition and performance of physical skills in children and youth. These developmentally based changes also influence the child's interaction with the physical and social environment. Therefore, models used to guide behavioral research on adults are not the most appropriate to use in studying children. To understand the child's involvement in physical activity, then, the sport and exercise scientist must understand these developmental changes and their ramifications.

Although interest in studying children's physical activity from a developmental behavioral science perspective has increased in recent years, few comprehensive reviews exist in the area, and interdisciplinary efforts are even less common. A need persists to review and integrate the behavioral science research on the child and physical activity. This volume is designed to help fill this void. Specifically, 11 reviews examine physical activity for children from historical, motor development, sociological, and psychological perspectives.

In chapter 1, sport historian David Wiggins provides the foundation for the remainder of the text by examining the rise of formal sport and informal play for North American children. He also presents an historical perspective on the interest of behavioral scientists in studying organized sport and play behavior of children and youth.

Gender differences in children's play and sport participation patterns are the focus of the second chapter by Crystal Branta, Mary Painter, and Joy Kiger. In addition to examining gender-linked sport and play participation patterns, the underlying explanations for these differences are discussed as well.

Children and the sport socialization process are the focus of the third chapter by sport sociologist, Jay Coakley. Areas addressed include factors affecting socialization into sport, the consequences of sport participation for children, and research on what children desire from sport. Coakley's chapter is followed by Dan Gould's review on attrition in organized sport for children. Both the descriptive and theoretical sport psychological research on this important topic are integrated into a model that serves to guide both future research and professional practice.

Chapters 5, 6, and 7 focus on central psychological concerns for those interested in physical activity for children: the development of children's self-esteem, the influence of adult behavior on children's psychological development, and the relationship between moral growth and physical activity participation. In particular, Maureen Weiss examines the development of children's self-esteem in physical activity settings and the relationship between self-esteem and physical achievement. In chapter 6, Thelma Horn discusses how teacher-coach behavior influences children's psychological development in physical activity environments. Then Brenda Bredemeier and David Shields consider moral growth through physical activity in chapter 7. These authors assimilate the latest theoretical and empirical research on this important topic by employing a structural/developmental approach.

The acquisition, development, and performance of children's motor skills are the major foci of chapters 8, 9, and 10. In chapter 8, Beverly Ulrich describes how children develop motor skills and factors that influence the development and performance of these skills. Memory development and its influence on sport skill acquisition are the topics of chapter 9, in which Jere Gallagher and Shirl Hoffman examine the empirical literature on related memory topics such as movement control, rapid decision making, and attention in children, as well as the use of this information in skill learning and performance situations. In chapter 10, Marjorie Woollacott, Bettina Debû, and Anne Shumway-Cook relate their systematic line of research on children's posture and balance control, with special attention placed on changes in motor coordination and sensory integration.

The final chapter of the text is unique in that Greg Reid discusses selected topics from the previous chapters by presenting both the behavioral and psychosocial variables related to physical activity in young handicapped performers. Emphasis is not only placed on the ramifications of these variables on handicapped performers, but also the theoretical advances that can be made by combining research on handicapped and normal children involved in physical activity settings.

In summary, this volume integrates the scholarly literature from a variety of behavioral science disciplines on the child and physical activity. In so doing, it summarizes what is known about this topic and holds implications for both scholars and practitioners alike. We hope that by providing summaries of the current state of knowledge in the area and suggesting blueprints for future study, new directions in pediatric behavioral science research will be initiated.

Daniel Gould
Maureen Weiss

# 1

# A History of Organized Play and Highly Competitive Sport for American Children

David K. Wiggins

Highly organized sport programs for American children had their beginnings in the last decade of the 19th century. Although children in this country had always participated in informal play activities and games among themselves or played on teams composed primarily of adults, large-scale, adult-directed sport programs were not established for youth (particularly boys) until the 1890s. The initial impetus for these programs came from the Young Men's Christian Association (YMCA), founded by evangelical Protestants in England in 1851 and transported to the United States prior to the Civil War. Partly in response to children's uncertain position in the increasingly urbanized and industrialized American society, the YMCA eventually reconsidered their traditional animosity toward sport for boys and began to organize leagues and to offer classes in physical culture.

During the first two decades of the 20th century, various schools, playgrounds, and national youth organizations such as the Boys Clubs and Boy

Scouts followed the YMCA's lead and also began providing recreational activities and organized sport for children. In the 1930s, however, professional recreation leaders and physical educators became disenchanted with various aspects of highly organized sport for children and relinquished their hold on the youth sport programs they had previously supported. As a result, after the 1940s highly organized sport for children left the educational context and was taken over by various volunteer youth groups in America. By the tumultuous 1960s, youth sport programs were being sponsored by professional sport organizations, Olympic committees, well-known business firms, colleges, and individual or community service groups. The last two decades have witnessed a continuing debate over the value of youth sport programs, with professional educators, medical doctors, and others arguing about the harmful effects or relative merits of sport competition for children. This ongoing debate has resulted in a voluminous number of research publications, the establishment of guidelines for youth sport coaches and parents, and the involvement of academicians in numerous youth sport projects over the last few years.

## MUSCULAR CHRISTIANITY AND THE YMCA

In the mid-19th century, American Protestants began to reexamine their traditional displeasure toward competitive sport for boys. Partly due to children's changing place in increasingly industrialized America, eastern aristocrats began to transform Protestant attitudes when they launched a crusade commonly referred to as Muscular Christianity. Newspaper editors and influential New England clergymen and writers tried to persuade eastern patricians of the compatibility of vigorous physical activity and spiritual sacredness. Thomas Wentworth Higginson, the most ardent supporter of Muscular Christianity, advocated a return to the Greek ideal of the harmonious development of mind, body, and spirit. Higginson, a Harvard Divinity School graduate who became actively involved in antislavery, women's suffrage, temperance, and other social reform movements, associated achievement with a vigorous childhood. He thus furnished a rationale for the advice-to-boys books that appeared in post–Civil War America (Lewis, 1966; Lucas, 1968; Rader, 1983).

The notion of Christian manliness as expressed by Higginson and other American intellectuals was often closely aligned with group loyalty, national pride, and patriotism. It also incorporated a number of character habits deemed suitable for American children. First, manly youth were to curtail their sexual appetites and refrain from practicing the "secret vice" of masturbation. This latter problem particularly troubled youth workers who feared that it robbed the body of needed energy and caused a myriad of other problems. Manly youth were also expected to be absolutely candid, to practice self-control, and to display no signs of affection or sentimentality. Perhaps more than anything else, manly youth were to be physically active and to develop their bodies to the fullest. Manly youth should discover the joys of rugged, outdoor recreation (Lewis, 1966; Lucas, 1968; Rader, 1983).

The most common mode of conveying Christian manliness to American boys was through sports fiction. *Tom Brown's School Days* (1857) was American boys' first important taste of the genre. Written by the lawyer Thomas Hughes and published in 1857, this masterpiece of Christian manliness was based on the author's experiences at the Rugby school during the years of the great headmaster, Thomas Arnold. *Tom Brown's School Days* was enormously popular and spawned a number of imitative works over the next few years such as G.W. Bankes's *A Day of My Life, or, Everyday Experiences at Eton* (1877); Bracebridge Hemyng's *Eton School Days* (1864); and Robert Grant's *Jack Hall, or The School Days of an American Boy* (1887). By the 1890s, a plethora of boys' sport novels began to appear in America that emphasized athletics even more than the previous works. Most notable among this group was Gilbert Patten's Frank Merriwell Stories, a series that began in 1896 and continued to appear in *Tip Top Weekly* for almost 20 years. Although he never explicitly espoused Christian doctrine, Patten nevertheless tried to convey to children that participation in vigorous physical activity contributed to character development and resulted in more material prosperity as an adult (Cutler, 1934; Evans, 1972).

Although sport fiction was the most popular vehicle for transmitting Muscular Christianity to American children, the YMCA became the most important institution associated with the movement. By the 1890s, the YMCA's traditional opposition to organized sport for children began to wane. To lure young men and boys into its organization, the YMCA broadened its program by offering classes in gymnastics and by establishing a competitive sport program (Boyer, 1978; Forbush, 1901; Forbush, 1904).

The YMCA's newly found interest in sport and physical culture resulted primarily from the efforts of one man, Luther Halsey Gulick. Born of missionary parents in Honolulu in 1865, Gulick believed strongly in the tenets of Muscular Christianity and spent a lifetime emphasizing physical and spiritual unity in man. Gulick officially became involved in the YMCA movement in 1887 when he was appointed the first secretary of the Physical Department of the International Committee of the YMCA of North America and also became instructor in the newly formed Department of Physical Training in the YMCA Training School in Springfield, Massachusetts. From 1889 to 1900, Gulick served as superintendent of the Physical Training Department (Dorgan, 1934; Forbush, 1901; Gerber, 1971).

Gulick's accomplishments while at the YMCA Training School were varied and many. He was the guiding force behind the development of a graduate diploma in physical education, a program that included courses in physiological psychology, the history and philosophy of physical education, anthropometry, and literature of physical education. He also organized, despite formidable opposition, a competitive sport program at the school for young men and adolescent boys. Perhaps most significantly, Gulick developed a pioneering course in the psychology of play. Students in the class were urged to experiment with new games and sports that were suitable for particular age groups. The invention of both basketball and volleyball emanated from Gulick's suggestions (Dorgan, 1934; Forbush, 1901; Gerber, 1971).

## THE EVOLUTIONARY THEORY OF PLAY

It is no surprise that Gulick initiated a course on the psychological aspects of play considering that he and his former mentor, G. Stanley Hall—the famous genetic psychologist from Clark University—had been developing an evolutionary theory of play. In fact, Gulick and Hall's play theory influenced Boy Work groups tremendously and had significant ramifications for using sport to promote social values during the first two decades of the 20th century. In their view, play survived because it re-created the physical processes through which humanity adapted to, and eventually dominated, the external world. The play activities of preadolescent children consisted of the same physical activities that had allowed primitive men and women to survive in a hostile environment. Therefore, such individual activities as running, chasing, and hurling objects toward a target were not just relics of the struggle for survival but instinctual acts requisite for the young child's healthy physical and psychic development. The more involved games of older children such as football, basketball, and baseball combined the primitive hunting instinct and the more recent instinct of cooperation. Vigorous physical activity that involved intimate contact between individuals was the primary agency in developing moral principles. Team sport, then, furnished an ideal occasion for adults to foster in boys the development of self-sacrifice, obedience, self-control, loyalty, and other qualities that were rapidly disappearing from modern society (Gulick, 1898, 1899).

## THE PUBLIC SCHOOL ATHLETIC LEAGUE
## AND THE PLAYGROUND MOVEMENT

Gulick had the opportunity to put his theory of play into practice in 1903 when he became the first Director of Physical Training in the public schools of New York City. Almost immediately upon his appointment, Gulick, with the assistance of James E. Sullivan, Secretary of the Amateur Athletic Union, and General George W. Wingate, a Civil War veteran who then served on the New York Board of Education, organized a massive athletic program for city school children called the Public School Athletic League (PSAL). Billed as the "World's Greatest Athletic Organization," PSAL was designed to allow every New York

City schoolchild an opportunity to participate in organized athletics. To guarantee that its philosophy of "Sports for All" was realized, the League had three separate forms of competition: class athletics, athletic badge tests, and interschool athletic competition. Competition in class athletics encouraged good students with limited athletic ability to participate with good athletes in various physical activities. Open to boys in the fifth to eighth grades, interested classes at each grade level performed pull-ups, the broad jump, and a dash. The three classes with the highest average for each event in each borough of New York City were retested by PSAL officials. If a class failed to equal or better its previous score, it was disqualified, and the class with the next lower average in that particular borough took its place. The class in each grade level with the highest average score for each event received a perpetual trophy that it kept for a year. An enormous number of boys participated in class athletics. In 1914 alone, 141,623 boys representing 8,049 classes took part in the competition (Gulick, 1905; Jable, 1979; Reeve, 1910; Wingate, 1908).

PSAL's athletic badge tests were just as important as class athletics in stimulating sport participation among New York City schoolchildren. To become eligible for an athletic badge, a boy had to do satisfactory work in the classroom and achieve the standards set by the league in jumping, running, and chinning events. The standards for boys under age 13 were running 8 3/5 seconds or less in the 60-yard dash, jumping a distance of 5 feet, 5 inches or more from a standing position, and doing four or more pull-ups. Boys over age 13 were expected to perform at a much higher level in each event (Gulick, 1905; Jable, 1979; Reeve, 1910; Wingate, 1908).

Highly skilled boys who found class athletics and the athletic badge tests unfulfilling took part in PSAL-sponsored interschool athletic competitions. These competitions, which took place on both the elementary and high school levels, culminated in city championships in a variety of different sports. In the beginning, PSAL emphasized sports with which the participants were already familiar. Competitions were held regularly in baseball, basketball, riflery, and track and field. By 1907, competitions were added in soccer, swimming, cross-country, lacrosse, tennis, roller skating, ice skating, and rowing (Gulick, 1905; Jable, 1979; Reeve, 1910; Wingate, 1908).

One of the special features of PSAL was the exercise and activity program it organized for girls in 1905. Under the leadership of Elizabeth Burchenal, the well-known physical educator who taught at both the Horace Mann School and Columbia University in New York City, the girls' branch of PSAL subscribed to Gulick's philosophy of inherent biological differences between the sexes. It sponsored games, walking events, and folk dancing for elementary-aged girls and certain track and field events for high school girls. The girls' branch emphasized group activities, forbidding individual and interschool competition in its program. Girls' teams could compete with one another only if they were located in the same school (Gerber, 1971; Gulick, 1905; Jable, 1979; Reeve, 1910; Wingate, 1908).

The philosophy of play espoused by Gulick and his followers was perhaps most clearly expressed in the early 20th-century movement for city playgrounds. Although philanthropic citizens and various charity groups had constructed play areas for children prior to the turn of the century, no large-scale playground system existed in America until 1903. In that year the voters of the Chicago South Park District passed a $5 million bond issue to open 10 parks. The parks were opened with the idea of promoting the health, morality, and sociability of people of all ages in Chicago. Realizing the need for trained leadership, the city commissioners employed the well-known physical educator E.B. DeGroot as Director of Gymnastics and Athletics. Each park was supervised by two instructors who, in most cases, had been trained in gymnastics and athletics at a college or normal school. Most of the centers in the South Park System had an outdoor area with a playground, swimming pool, and facilities for soccer, hockey, ice skating, football, and baseball. Also included in many programs were physical training activities; parties; banquets; lectures on public issues and child welfare; and theatrical, orchestral, and dance programs (Kadjielski, 1977; Mergen, 1975; Rainwater, 1922).

Perhaps the key event in the push for playgrounds was the establishment in 1906 of the Playground Association of America, an organization founded largely through the efforts of Gulick and Dr. Henry Curtis, a pioneer playground worker from Washington, DC. From the beginning, this organization was instrumental in arousing public interest in the right of children to play. In 1907, it began publishing an official monthly magazine called *The Playground*. Three years later, a special committee within the organization prepared a book entitled *The Normal Course in Play*, which outlined for the first time scientific training for recreation workers (Hetherington, 1910). The organization also served as a clearinghouse, accumulating data from all over the United States and disseminating this information to interested recreation leaders. In addition, it sponsored workshops to train play leaders and to improve the quality of recreation leadership (Curtis, 1917; Rainwater, 1922).

The success of the Playground Association resulted primarily from its skilled leadership. Joseph Lee—a pioneer social worker, philanthropist, and author of one of the most influential books on play, *Play in Education* (1916)—became president of the organization in 1910, and another social worker, Howard Broucher, became secretary. Through their direction and financial support, these two men did much to advance the growth of playgrounds and public recreation. Besides Gulick, who served as the organization's president for 3 years, many other prominent physical educators assumed leadership roles in the Playground Association, including George W. Ehler, Joseph E. Raycroft, George Meylan, George Fisher, James McCurdy, and Clark Hetherington. Hetherington, the author of the Association's book *The Normal Course in Play* (1910), was perhaps most active in the promotion of playgrounds and recreation.

A graduate of Stanford University and a student of G. Stanley Hall at Clark University for 2 years, Hetherington was profoundly interested in children's play. To Hetherington, play was a child's chief business in life, play was superior to work as a developer of the nervous system, and play was an educational endeavor. Hetherington had many opportunities to practice this theory of play, but his most noteworthy accomplishment was the establishment of the Demonstration Play School at the University of California, Berkeley, in 1913. A program established for children between 4 and 12 years old, the play school lasted 3 hours a day for 6 weeks during the university's regular summer session. Hetherington's aim in founding the play school was to provide children with an opportunity to develop themselves physically, socially, emotionally, and morally. In tune with a progressive educational curriculum, Hetherington devised a system that incorporated eight types of activities, including:

• economic activities, such as bookkeeping and banking;

• vocal and linguistic activities such as storytelling;

• social activities in which children learned acceptable democratic values;

• rhythmic and musical activities including the use of premusical instruments;

• dramatic activities including plays and pageants;

• environmental activities such as excursions;

• manipulative and manual activities like arts and crafts; and

• hip-muscle activities such as dancing, games, gymnastics, and competitive athletics.

The demonstration play school was quite successful. It became a model school and was studied by educators from around the country until it was forced to close in 1934 because of lack of funds (Gerber, 1971).

## LITTLE LEAGUE BASEBALL AND THE ORGANIZATION OF COMPETITIVE SPORT PROGRAMS

Although many American children experienced organized play and competitive athletics for the first time on city playgrounds and in such innovative institutions as Hetherington's demonstrative school, it was not until the 1920s and 1930s that highly organized sport programs for children were established outside the educational realm. These programs emerged mainly because of the adults' continued interest in the welfare of children and the fact that sport was becoming enormously popular in American society. One of the first programs established was the Junior Baseball Tournament held in Cincinnati for boys under age 13. Organized by the Cincinnati Community Service in 1924, this tournament involved 84 teams and received hearty endorsement from the commissioner of major league baseball, Judge Kenesaw M. Landis. In 1927, Denver began a tackle football program for boys under age 12. The *Los Angeles Times* organized its Junior Pentathlon in 1928. Two years later the Catholic Youth Organization founded its junior tennis program under the auspices of the Southern California Tennis Association, and the Pop Warner football began as a four-team league in Philadelphia. In 1936, the Milwaukee Recreation Department organized its "Stars of Yesterday" baseball program for boys under 15.

Most importantly, Little League baseball was founded by Carl Stotz in Williamsport, Pennsylvania in 1939. Designed to develop "qualities of citizenship, sportsmanship, and manhood" in boys 8 to 12 years old, Little League baseball attracted only local attention during its first several years of existence. The league slowly expanded and by 1947 began sponsoring its now famous Little League World Series (Berryman, 1975; Cloyd, 1952; Monroe, 1946; Paxton, 1949).

Ironically, these programs were being established at about the same time professional educators began to discourage highly competitive sport for young children in and outside the school setting. Between approximately 1930 and the first half of the 1950s, professional educators consistently condemned competitive sport for elementary aged children. For instance, Elmer D. Mitchell, the well-known physical educator from the University of Michigan, was one of the first professionals to express his displeasure of competitive sport programs for schoolchildren. In 1932, he urged junior high schools to drop interscholastic athletic competition and to adopt an intramural or "Sport Days" program. Competitive sport programs for children, wrote Mitchell, caused "premature specialization," encouraged harmful newspaper notoriety, and unduly harmed the participants physically and emotionally (Mitchell, 1932, p. 22).

Six years after Mitchell's editorial, the American Association for Health, Physical Education, and Recreation (AAHPER, 1938) passed a resolution at their convention in Atlanta condemning highly competitive sport for elementary schoolchildren. In 1938 and 1946, the Society of State Directors of Physical and Health Education proclaimed that interschool athletic leagues should be confined to senior high schools and had no place in elementary or junior high schools. They specifically discouraged championship games, all-star teams, and traveling (Lowman, 1947; Moss & Orion, 1939). AAHPER passed another resolution in 1947 opposing interscholastic competition for children below the ninth grade. That same year it made a joint policy statement with the National Federation of High School Athletic Associations (NFHSAA) recommending that intramural programs be developed at the elementary school level (AAHPER, 1947). In 1949, the Joint Committee on Athletic Competition for Children of Elementary and Junior High School Age recommended that highly competitive sport programs for children be abolished. This group—which was made up of representatives from AAHPER, the Society of State Directors of Health, Physical Education and Recreation, the Department of Elementary School Principals, the National Education Association, and the National Council of State Consultants in Elementary Education—made an extensive policy statement directed at community groups as well as school programs (AAHPER, 1952). Finally, in the early 1950s AAHPER, the National Conference of Program Planning in Games and Sport for Boys of School Age, the National Conference on Physical Education for Children of Elementary School Age, and the National Recreation Congress all made statements condemning competitive sport programs for children (AAHPER, 1952; National Recreation Congress, 1952; Wayman, 1950).

The policy statements of various educational groups were responsible for the discontinuance of some interschool competitive sport programs at the elementary age level. The recommendations hardly affected, however, children's sport programs outside the school setting. In fact, between the founding of Little League baseball in 1939 and the latter half of the 1960s, a plethora of competitive sport programs for children was established, and already existing programs continued to flourish. These programs were sponsored by several different interest groups, including religious organizations, community recreation departments, community service clubs, nonprofit community agencies, national youth sport agencies, business firms, Olympic committees, professional sport organizations, and colleges.

In 1947, for example, the U.S. Chamber of Commerce began their sponsorship of children's sports (Berryman, 1975). Three years later, Jay Archer, the executive director of the Catholic Youth Center, founded Biddy Basketball in Scranton, Pennsylvania (Archer, 1950). Organized for boys and girls 8 to 11 years old, this sport program aimed to develop in children "a love for the game of basketball . . . and a fine sense of sportsmanship" (p. 270). In 1952, Pony Baseball was incorporated as a nonprofit organization (Berryman, 1975). Ten years later the American Youth Soccer Association was founded in Torrance, California, a sport program with nearly 200,000 participants by 1977 (Berryman, 1975). In 1967, the Soccer Association for Youth was established in Ohio (Berryman, 1975). That same year, the Amateur Fencers League of America incorporated their Junior Olympic Fencing Program (Berryman, 1975). In 1969, the National Youth Sports Program (NYSP) was established to give disadvantaged children 10 to 16 years old an opportunity to participate in competitive sport. Cosponsored by the Office of Community Services and the National Collegiate Athletic Association (NCAA), the NYSP projects are conducted during the summer months on nearly 146 college campuses across the country (NCAA, 1985).

Another important youth sport organization founded in the 1960s was the Special Olympics. Eunice Kennedy Shriver began a summer camp in Maryland in June, 1963 for mentally retarded individuals primarily designed to test the capabilities of the mentally retarded in a number of sport activities. Over the next 5 years hundreds of communities and private organizations established similar camps for the mentally retarded. In July, 1968 the Kennedy Foundation and the Chicago Park District held the first International Special Olympics at Chicago's Soldier Field for some 1,000 mentally retarded children from 26 states and Canada. Five months later, the Special Olympics was established as a nonprofit charitable organization under the laws of the District of Columbia. Almost immediately the Council for Exceptional Children, the National Association for Retarded Citizens, and the American Association on Mental Deficiencies pledged their support for this first systematic effort to provide athletic competition for the mentally retarded. By the beginning of 1970, all 50 states, the District of Columbia, and Canada had Special Olympics organizations and state directors (Special Olympics, n.d.).

The establishment of new programs and increased participation of children in competitive sport during the middle decades of the 20th century resulted from several factors. Part of the reason was the continued belief of many parents and guardians that the benefits gleaned from competitive sport participation far outweighed any negative consequences. Implicit in most adult-directed programs by this time was the belief that competitive sport participation contributed positively to a child's physical fitness, sense of sportsmanship, and overall character development. Also contributing to the growth of children's sport during this period were the increasing amount of media coverage given to top-level amateur and professional sport and the constant glory heaped on star athletes. Children and their parents could not help but be impressed by all the money and attention lavished on big-time athletes. Early involvement in competitive sport might put children on a similar path to fame and fortune. The growth of children's sport might also be due to the increased involvement of women in the work force, greater accessibility of youth sport programs, and the changing lifestyle of many adults.

## THE GIRLS' MOVEMENT IN YOUTH SPORTS

The increased involvement of children in competitive athletics during the middle of the 20th century was truly significant but not as important as the events and changes that took place in youth sport during the 1970s. In fact, this decade can rightfully be termed the watershed in the history of children's sport. Perhaps the most publicized event that took place during this period was the desegregation of Little League baseball. Growing out of the campaign waged against sexual discrimination in all aspects of American life during the early 1970s, the national Little Leagues' ban against participation by girls was challenged by individual girls and parents for the first time in 1973. In May of that year, Jenny Fuller, a young ball player from California, wrote a letter to President Nixon complaining that she was not given an opportunity to play for her local Little League team. She received a response from the Office of Civil Rights explaining that it was in the process of establishing policies to deal with such discriminatory practices. At about the same time, other young girls unsuccessfully attempted to play for local Little League teams in Portland, Oregon; Fairfax County, Virginia; Ypsilanti, Michigan; and Hoboken, New Jersey (Jennings, 1981).

In those cases where girls attempted to integrate local teams, the national Little League organization threatened to withdraw the local league's charter. Not willing to sacrifice its programs for the benefit of a few individual girls, most local officials followed the dictates of the national Little League organization and prohibited girls from participating in their league. The one exception to this rule occurred in Hoboken, New Jersey where Maria Pepe's unsuccessful attempt to play on a local team culminated in an investigation by the New Jersey Division of Civil Rights and ultimately in the desegregation of Little League baseball. At the request of the Essex Chapter of the National Organization for Women (NOW), the Civil Rights Division conducted a hearing in November, 1973 on behalf of Pepe and other girls between 8 and 12 years old. During 6 days of deliberation, the Little League attempted to rationalize its position by having expert witnesses present scientific evidence confirming that highly competitive athletics was too hazardous for girls both physiologically and psychologically. Dr. Thomas Johnson argued that children might develop psychological problems if they were forced to integrate because young girls preferred to keep company with other young girls and young boys with other young boys. Dr. Creighton Hale, an expert in physiology and executive vice-president of the national Little League, cited many research studies that indicated that girls' bones were developmentally weaker than those of boys. He also contended that girls stood a serious chance of harming their breasts during strenuous athletic participation. Hale pointed out, moreover, that a "substantial body" of the medical profession was convinced that injuries to the breasts caused cancer (Jennings, 1981).

The Civil Rights Division countered with its own expert testimony. Dr. Antonio Giancotti rebutted Dr. Johnson's previous assertions by stating that integrated sport activities for preadolescent children would, in his opinion, contribute to positive mental health. Dr. Joseph Torg, a pediatric-orthopedic surgeon, testified that 8- to 12-year-old girls were more likely to have stronger bones than boys the same age. He also chided Dr. Hale for basing his testimony upon studies that examined the bones of adult cadavers rather than those of children (Jennings, 1981).

The Civil Rights Division ruled that Little League baseball's refusal to allow girls into its program violated both state and federal laws. Sylvia Pressler, the Division's hearing officer, stated that she was convinced that performance differences of children between 8 and 12 years old were founded on an individual basis, not on a sexual class basis. Because Little League baseball was a federally chartered organization and had submitted to the New Jersey Division of Civil Rights, Pressler saw no reason that national policy prohibiting sexual discrimination should not be enforced. It was obvious from Pressler's ruling that if the decision was upheld by Superior Courts, Little League baseball would be forced to allow girls to participate in its programs (Jennings, 1981).

Little League baseball challenged Pressler's ruling, appealing to the appellation division of New Jersey's Superior Court in late March, 1974. The Little League challenged the Civil Rights Division ruling, insisted that its Federal Charter specifically banned girls, and stated that New Jersey Statutes allowed only boys to participate on its local teams. To its consternation, the Little League lost its appeal. On March 29, 1974, the state Superior Court decided that a local league chartered by Little League, Inc. was a "place of public accommodation" and therefore not exempt from Federal Legislation against sexual discrimination (Jennings, 1981, p. 85).

Although girls had legally won the right to participate in Little League baseball, the desegregation of teams in New Jersey and elsewhere occurred sporadically and amidst continuing opposition. Subtle discrimination existed even in those leagues where girls supposedly enjoyed equal opportunities. A local league in Romulus, Michigan, for example, made it mandatory in 1975 that every player wear a cup and athletic supporter. In Union, New Jersey girls could participate in tryouts only if a parent or guardian was in attendance. Some Little League officials and parents still worried that girls risked damaging their vital parts and suffered morally by participating in nonsegregated competitive sport. Some people believed that an injury might entice coaches to clutch a girl while giving first aid (Jennings, 1981).

The fact that desegregation of Little League baseball has been painstakingly slow does not minimize the importance of the landmark decision of the New Jersey Supreme Court. Girls can now choose to be participants in Little League baseball rather than merely spectators. This, in and of itself, is of monumental importance to young girls who can now participate in this country's national pastime and in one of youth sports oldest and most prestigious programs.

## THE GROWTH OF YOUTH SPORTS: INSTITUTES, CONFERENCES, AND COACHING EDUCATION PROGRAMS

The 1970s witnessed not only the desegregation of Little League baseball but also a change in attitude toward children's sport by professional educators, administrators, and physicians. An indication of the more conciliatory position taken by these groups was the increasing number of professional meetings that included papers, sessions, and symposiums devoted to various aspects of youth sports. The American Alliance for Health, Physical Education, Recreation, and Dance (AAHPERD), the National Association for Physical Education in Higher Education (NAPEHE), and other national organizations invariably included topics dealing with children's sports in their annual conference program. Evidence that professionals were altering their position was also seen in the number of conferences organized during this decade that dealt exclusively with the research being carried out on children's sport participation. In 1973, for instance, a conference entitled "The Child in Sport and Physical Activity" was held at Queens University in Kingston, Ontario, Canada. Some of the most respected researchers in North America presented papers on youth sport from a physiological, medical, motor development, psychological, sociological, and motor learning perspective. Seven of those papers comprise a book edited by J.G. Albinson and G.M. Andrew, the organizers of the conference and physical educators from Queens University (Albinson & Andrew, 1976). In March, 1977, a similar conference entitled "Contemporary Research on Youth Sports" was held at the University of Washington. Sponsored jointly by the Departments of Psychology and Physical Education at the University of Washington, the conference was designed to give academicians from North America an opportunity to exchange research ideas in the area of youth sports and to discuss possible directions for future research. The conference, which included as participants such notable scholars as Robert Malina, Lawrence Rarick, Jerry Thomas, Glyn Roberts, Tara Scanlan, and Mike Passer, touched on subjects ranging from "Significant Others and Sport Socialization of the Handicapped Child" to "Coaching Behaviors in Little League Baseball." An outgrowth of the conference was publication of the research papers in a book edited by Frank Smoll and Ronald Smith entitled *Psychological Perspectives in Youth Sports* (1978).

The more balanced approach taken by professionals during the 1970s was further evidenced by the guidelines and large-scale legislative studies completed on children's sport. In 1976, AAHPERD established the National Association for Sport and Physical Education Youth Sports Task Force to examine the current status of children's sport and to offer suggestions concerning youth sport programs. Made up of experts from the medical, recreational, and physical education professions, the work of the task force was summarized in a book edited by Rainer Martens and Vern Seefeldt entitled *Guidelines for Children's Sports* (1979). In effect, the task force recognized the important role of sport in many children's lives and how essential it was that youth sport leaders provide "safe, satisfying, and beneficial experiences" for their young charges. To guarantee that children were provided with a pleasurable and meaningful sport experience, the well-known "Bill of Rights for Young Athletes" was prepared.

Easily the most ambitious project undertaken on children's sport during the 1970s was Michigan's Joint Legislative Study Committee on Youth Sports Program. In the winter of 1975, this special six-member committee was established to investigate and study the state's youth sport activities programs. To assist them in their study, the committee immediately contacted representatives from Michigan State University, Northern Michigan University, the University of Michigan, and Wayne State University. During April and May, 1975 these representatives held several meetings on the subject, and after much discussion they submitted a research proposal to the Joint Legislative Study Committee. The proposal described a longitudinal study that was designed to assess the impact that certain competitive sport programs had on the development of children between 5 and 17. Specific information was sought on both the beneficial and harmful effects that the aforementioned programs had on the physical, psychological, and social development of preadolescent children (Joint Legislative Study [JLS], 1976).

The research proposal was accepted by the Joint Legislative Study Committee in July, 1978, and Phase 1 of the program was implemented immediately. The primary purpose of Phase 1, which lasted through October, 1976, was to determine the extent of participation of Michigan schoolchildren in recreational activities and in competitive sport programs within and outside the school system. Phase 2 of the program examined issues critical to the welfare of children in competitive sport programs. Those children who did not participate in competitive sport, along with their parents, were also asked to complete a questionnaire pertaining to their views on youth sport. The third and final phase of the program attempted to determine, among other things, the seat of administrative control over youth sports in Michigan and the qualifications of coaches directing competitive athletics for children (JLS, 1978a, 1978b).

The results of all three phases were presented to the Legislative Study Committee by November, 1978. The data indicated that the majority of children in Michigan received their initial exposure to competitive sport through recreational and non-school-sponsored programs. Children, both male and female, engaged in youth sport programs primarily for enjoyment and to increase skill level. The coaches, administrators, and other leaders indicated that they participated in youth sports either because their children were involved in the program or because they possessed expertise needed by the particular organization. One of the overriding problems in Michigan was the lack of good interpersonal relationships between the various groups involved in youth sport programs (JLS, 1978a, 1978b).

The most visible and far-reaching outcome of the 3-year legislative study was the establishment of the Youth Sports Institute (YSI) at Michigan State University in the summer of 1978. Under the directorship of Professor Vern Seefeldt, the institute was founded to conduct scientific research on children's sport participation; to provide in-service education for volunteer coaches; and to furnish educational materials for parents, volunteer coaches, and officials involved in youth sport programs. Since its founding, the institute has held numerous workshops and clinics for coaches, officials, and administrators. It has also published a number of pamphlets and books dealing with various aspects of youth sports, including *Motivating Young Athletes* (Gould, 1980); *A Winning Philosophy for Youth Sports Programs* (Seefeldt, Smoll, Smith, & Gould, 1981); and *Improving Relationship Skills in Youth Sport Coaches*

(Smoll & Smith, 1979). The institute also publishes a newsletter entitled *Spotlight in Youth Sports*, a quarterly communication that is distributed free to people involved in Michigan youth sport programs.

The establishment of the Youth Sport Institute at Michigan State took place at about the same time as the founding of two other youth sport organizations, the National Council of Youth Sports Directors (NCYSD) and the North American Youth Sport Institute (NAYSI). NCYSD, an organization established for the purpose of mutual cooperation and sharing of information between executives of youth sport programs, held its first meeting in Chicago in 1978. Originally sponsored in cooperation with the Athletic Institute, NCYSD became an independent organization in 1979 and has as its members "full-time professional staff persons of amateur, non-profit organizations who direct a national program involving youth sports." Some of the organizations represented in NCYSD are AAU Junior Olympics, The American Amateur Baseball Congress, the American Youth Soccer Organization, Babe Ruth Baseball, the National Federation of State High School Associations, the National Junior Tennis League, Pop Warner Football, the U.S. Field Hockey Association, U.S.A. Wrestling, and the YMCA (NCYSD, n.d.).

NAYSI was founded in November, 1979 in Kernersville, North Carolina as a private youth sport organization following several futile attempts to secure funding from the business community. NAYSI conducts workshops and clinics for youth sport coaches, sponsors research and evaluation projects, organizes local advisory bodies that help plan youth sport programs, and does consulting work for various youth sport agencies. NAYSI also produced a magazine entitled *Sport Scene*, a quarterly publication that included articles on the latest scientific research, training aids, new program ideas, suggestions on skill development, management procedures, and conference proceedings (Cox, 1982).

Significantly, both NAYSI and YSI have devoted much of their time to educating youth sport coaches, but they are not the only ones that have been actively involved in this type of work. In fact, over the last several years a number of programs have been established specifically to educate those people involved in coaching young athletes. Most people associated with youth sport programs now recognize that competent and well-qualified coaches are essential if a boy or girl is to have a positive athletic experience.

Two of the programs involved in educating youth sport coaches are the YMCA Youth Sports Training Programs and the National Youth Sports Coaches Association (NYSCA). The latter program is perhaps the most noteworthy. Organized in January 1981, NYSCA is the officially endorsed program of the National Recreation and Parks Association. The program receives its primary support from memberships of official NYSCA training centers and the NYSCA Volunteer Coaches Certification Program. Its major purposes are to train and certify youth sport coaches; to educate the general public about youth sport programs; to encourage high standards of sportsmanship among those involved in youth sports; to promote better understanding among athletes, the general public, and the administrators of youth sports programs; and to conduct and disseminate research dealing with all aspects of youth sports. Like many of the other organizations, NYSCA publishes its own quarterly newsletter entitled *Youth Sport Coach* (NYSCA, n.d.).

The most recognizable coaching education program in the United States is the American Coaching Effectiveness Program (ACEP). The origin of ACEP can be traced to 1974 when Bryant J. Cratty, a well-known sport psychologist from the University of California at Los Angeles, and Rainer Martens, an equally acclaimed sport psychologist from the University of Illinois, were invited by the Soviet Union Sport Committee to spend 2 weeks visiting the sport institutes in Leningrad, Tblisi, and Moscow. During the visit Professor Martens became well acquainted with Dr. Yuri Hanin, a senior researcher in sport psychology at the Research Institute of Physical Culture in Leningrad. Over the next 3 years the two sport scientists maintained a continuing correspondence centering primarily around the question of bridging the communication gap between sport psychologists and coaches and athletes in the field. Hanin told Martens that the most puzzling aspect of sport psychology in North America was researchers' failure to assist athletes and coaches in their work. Hanin related that the dissemination of sport psychology research to coaches and athletes in the field had increased substantially in his country over the last few years. Publication of research in the monthly *Theory of Practice of Physical Culture Journal* and in specialized yearbooks kept Soviet sport teams up-to-date on the latest scientific information (Hanin & Martens, 1978).

Martens was determined to establish the same kind of communication between sport scientists and coaches in this country and began by establishing a newsletter especially for youth sport coaches entitled *Sportsline* in 1979. Published by the Office of Youth Sports at the University of Illinois, *Sportsline* focused on the scientific principles of coaching. The latest research findings from such disciplinary areas as sport psychology, sport sociology, exercise physiology, sport biomechanics, and motor learning and development, were made available to coaches through this quarterly newsletter (Office of Youth Sports [OYS], 1979a).

The launching of *Sportsline* set the stage for a series of summer short courses offered by the Office of Youth Sports during June and July, 1979. Designed especially for youth sport coaches and administrators, the four 1-week courses touched upon some of the prominent issues in children's sport from both theoretical and practical perspectives. Each course was taught by a prominent individual who was well versed in his particular field and who had extensive experience in youth sport programs. Martens taught one course that focused on such things as the competitive process and prominent psychological issues in youth sports. Dan Foster, a certified athletic trainer from the University of Iowa, taught a course in sports medicine, examining in particular the traumatic injuries that occur in children's sport. Joseph Pechinsk, an exercise physiologist from the University of Maine, focused on the value of physiological knowledge for youth sport coaches in his course. Robert Christina, the well-known motor learning specialist from Pennsylvania State University, taught the fourth and final course that centered on instructional methods for youth coaches (OYS, 1979b).

The summer short courses offered by the Office of Youth Sports, along with a subsequent coaching effectiveness program implemented by U.S.A. Wrestling, were the forerunners of the ACEP officially founded by Martens in 1980. Perhaps the most comprehensive coaching education program available today, ACEP emerged only after careful scrutiny of existing programs and hundreds of interviews with coaches around the country. ACEP gives coaches a general understanding of sports medicine and science and instructs them in the most appropriate ways to teach the fundamentals and techniques of their particular sport. The program involves three primary levels: Level 1 teaches the basic concepts essential for all youth sport coaches; Level 2 furnishes additional information on each of the topics covered in the first level; and Level 3 is geared toward those coaches involved with top-level athletes. In addition, ACEP offers Leadership Training Seminars for youth sport administrators interested in making ACEP a part of their program. In sum, ACEP is enormously popular, having been adopted by a large number of international, national, state, and local organizations (ACEP, 1984).

## THE GROWTH OF YOUTH SPORTS:
## PUBLICATIONS AND RESEARCH

One of the most conspicuous developments over the last 15 years has been the publication of a voluminous amount of popular literature and research studies dealing with various aspects of youth sports. Hundreds of articles, either praising or condemning highly competitive sport programs for children, have appeared in such journals as *Sports Illustrated, Look, Life, Changing Times, Parent's Magazine, Todays Health, New York Times Magazine, Better Homes and Gardens, U.S. News and World Report, Ladies Home Journal,* and *The Atlantic Monthly*. The authors of these particular articles have ranged from concerned parents and senior staff writers to famous sport personalities like Fran Tarkenton, Bob Feller, and Robin Roberts (Feller, 1956; Roberts, 1975; Tarkenton, 1970; Underwood, 1975).

Perhaps more enlightening than the aforementioned works is a number of reminiscences of Little League baseball written mainly by parents and former players. For instance, Al Rosen, a former major league ball player, discusses the complexities of Little League baseball in his book, *Baseball and Your Boy* (1967). Rosen views Little League baseball as an activity for children that is by necessity supervised by adults. Rosen asserts that a boy will profit from participation in Little League baseball if his parents are supportive and understanding and if his coach is enthusiastic as well as competent. In their book

*Laughing and Crying with Little League* (1972), Catherine and Loren Broadus, the parents of three former Little League baseball players, discuss the hardships faced by coaches, officials, and parents involved in youth sports. The authors also provide practical solutions to problems commonly associated with children's competitive sport programs. In a slightly different vein, Martin Ralbovsky's *Destiny's Darlings* (1974) tells the story of the Schenectady Little League team that won the world championship in 1954. Ralbovsky, a writer for the *New York Times* who grew up in Schenectady, interviewed nine players and the manager of the team 20 years later to assess what winning the championship had meant to them. Their story, unfortunately, is generally one of frustration and disillusionment.

A number of books has also been written over the last 15 years, in addition to the ones previously mentioned, that are devoted exclusively to coaching youth sports. These works range from popular types of coaching manuals to more scholarly oriented publications. Thomas Johnson, a former Little League player, coach, and official, wrote one of the first books on coaching youth sports. In a 1973 work entitled *My Coach Says . . .* , Johnson provides an excellent guide for coaches involved in youth sport programs and offers valuable suggestions for dealing with problem players. Richard Bluth's monograph, *Coaching Youth League Baseball* (1975), offers a great deal of information for coaches involved with youth baseball players. Bluth describes the proper techniques involved in throwing, pitching, hitting, fielding, baserunning, and discusses team player selection. Jerry Thomas's edited book, *Youth Sports Guide for Coaches and Parents* (1977), was the first coaching manual published by a national youth sport association. Produced by AAHPERD, this guide covers such topics as physiological development, psychological issues, instructional strategies, motivating young athletes, managing a team, and the issue of winning and losing. Perhaps the most comprehensive book on the subject is *Coaching Young Athletes* (1981), a publication edited by Rainer Martens, Robert W. Christina, John S. Harvey, Jr., and Brian J. Sharkey. The book covers the various ramifications of youth sport coaching from philosophical, psychological, pedagogical, physiological, and sport medicine perspectives.

In addition to the aforementioned works, a myriad of research studies has been published on youth sports over the last several years. The studies have been completed by academicians from a variety of disciplinary perspectives and have ranged from research dealing with psychological stress on young athletes to the physiological stress on young athletes to the physiological effects of youth sport participation. One encouraging research trend is the fact that many scholars have established a specific line of inquiry and have designed large-scale longitudinal projects dealing with youth sport participation. Nowhere is this more evident than in the research completed in the subdisciplinary area of sport psychology. For instance, Ron Smith and Frank Smoll, two well-known academicians from the University of Washington, have been involved the last number of years in examining the leadership behaviors of youth sport coaches and in focusing on the psychological correlates of children's motor development. The two scholars have developed a psychologically oriented, nationally recognized training program for youth sport coaches, called Coach Effectiveness Training (Smith & Smoll, 1982a, 1982b; Smith, Smoll, & Curtis, 1979; Smith, Smoll, & Hunt, 1977; Smoll & Smith, 1980).

A multitude of works has been published on youth sports during the last few years that are not easily classified but should be mentioned because of their importance to the field. Certainly one of the more important books is Rainer Martens's *Joy and Sadness in Children's Sports* (1978), a thoroughly comprehensive work that contains 25 articles on children's sport. Terry Orlick and Cal Botterill discuss how important the process of competition is for young athletes in their 1976 book, *Every Kid Can Win*. One of the joys of this book is that readers will find themselves viewing sport from their own childhood experiences. In 1978 Richard Magill, Michael Ash, and Frank Smoll edited *Children in Sport: A Contemporary Anthology*, a book that examines youth sports from a variety of perspectives. Some of the most respected sport scientists contributed papers on such topics as children's socialization into sports, anatomical and physiological issues in youth sports, and psychological and moral concerns in children's sport. Finally, Maureen Weiss and Daniel Gould (1986) edited a volume of the proceedings of the 1984 Olympic Scientific Congress titled *Sport for Children and Youths*. In this text scholars from around the world examine critical issues such as when children should begin competing, perceptions of stress, injuries in youth sports, and game modification.

Many more publications on youth sport exist that are worthy of mention. Thomas Tutko and William Bruns's *Winning is Everything and Other American Myths* (1976), David Voigt's *A Little League Journal* (1974), and Richard Cox's *Educating Youth Sports Coaches: Solutions to a National Dilemma* (1982) are just a few works that come to mind. Suffice it to say that the involvement of children in highly competitive sport has increased dramatically over the last 80 years or so. Children of both sexes can now participate in almost any sport and can be assured, in most cases, that they will receive quality instruction from concerned coaches. Although some Americans continue to approach youth sport programs with skepticism, an ever-increasing belief exists that, if properly organized, children's highly competitive sport programs can be a very positive and worthwhile experience. The traditional animosity toward children's competitive sport that existed during the latter half of the 19th century has now given way to a multitude of youth sport programs sponsored by a variety of different organizations. The growth of these programs has been accompanied by an increase in the literature on children's sport, the organization of youth sport institutes, the development of youth sport coaching programs, and the staging of symposiums and conferences devoted to children's sport. Obviously, youth sport programs in America are not only tolerated but deemed necessary for the overall development of the child. This is a far cry from the attitude of most Americans nearly a hundred years ago.

## REFERENCES

Albinson, J.G., & Andrew, G.M. (Eds.). (1976). *Child in sport and physical activity*. Baltimore: University Park Press.

American Alliance for Health, Physical Education, and Recreation. (1938). Two important resolutions. *Journal of Health and Physical Education, 9*, 488–489.

American Alliance for Health, Physical Education, and Recreation. (1947). *Cardinal athletic principles*. Washington, DC: Author and National Education Association.

American Alliance for Health, Physical Education, and Recreation. (1952). *Desirable athletic competition for children*. Washington, DC: Author.

American Coaching Effectiveness Program. (1984). *Brochure*. Champaign, IL: Human Kinetics.

Archer, J. (1950). Questions about biddy basketball. *Recreation, 44*, 270.

Bankes, G.W. (1877). *A day of my life; or, everyday experiences at Eton*. London: Stanley Paul.

Berryman, J.W. (1975). From the cradle to the playing field: America's emphasis on highly competitive sports for pre-adolescent boys. *Journal of Sport History, 2*, 112–131.

Bluth, R. (1975). *Coaching youth league baseball*. Chicago: The Athletic Institute.

Boyer, P. (1978). *Urban masses and moral order in America, 1820–1920*. Cambridge, MA: Harvard University Press.

Broadus, C., & Broadus, L. (1972). *Laughing and crying with Little League*. New York: Harper and Row.

Cloyd, J. (1952). Gangway for the mighty midgets. *American Magazine, 154*, 28–29, 83–85.

Cox, R. (Ed.). (1982). *Educating youth sport coaches: Solutions to a national dilemma*. Reston, VA: American Alliance for Health, Physical Education, Recreation, and Dance.

Curtis, H.S. (1917). *The play movement and its significance*. New York: Macmillan.

Cutler, J.L. (1934). *Gilbert Patten and his Frank Merriwell saga*. Orono: University of Maine Studies.

Dorgan, E.J. (1934). *Luther Halsey Gulick, 1865–1918*. New York: Teachers College, Columbia University.

Evans, W. (1972). The all American boys: A study of boys' sport fiction. *Journal of Popular Culture, 6*, 104–121.

Feller, B. (1956, August). Don't knock Little Leagues. *Colliers,* pp. 78–81.

Forbush, W.B. (1901). *The boy problem: A study in social pedagogy.* Boston: Pilgrim Press.

Forbush, W.B. (1904). Can the Y.M.C.A. do all the street boys' work? *Work With Boys, 4,* 182.

Gerber, E.W. (1971). *Innovators and institutions in physical education.* Philadelphia: Lea & Febiger.

Gould, D. (1980). *Motivating young athletes.* East Lansing, MI: Youth Sports Institute.

Grant, R. (1887). *Jack Hall, or the school days of an American boy.* New York: Scribner's.

Gulick, L.H. (1898). Physical aspects of group games. *Popular Science Monthly, 53,* 793–805.

Gulick, L.H. (1899). Psychological, pedagogical, and religious aspects of group games. *Pedagogical Seminary, 6,* 144.

Gulick, L.H. (1905). How to start a public schools athletic league. *Work With Boys, 4,* 232–235.

Hanin, Y., & Martens, R. (1978). Sport psychology in the U.S.S.R. *Coaching Review, 5,* 32–41.

Hemyng, B. (1864). *Eton school days.* London: Hutchinson.

Hetherington, C.W. (1910). *A normal course in play.* New York: Playground Association of America.

Hughes, T. (1857). *Tom Brown's school days.* New York: Harper and Brothers.

Jable, J.T. (1979). The Public School Athletic League of New York City: Organized athletics for city schoolchildren, 1903–1914. In W.M. Ladd & A. Lumpkin (Eds.), *Sport in American education: History and perspective* (pp. ix–18). Washington, DC: American Alliance for Health, Physical Education, Recreation, and Dance.

Jennings, S.E. (1981). As American as hot dogs, apple pie and Chevrolet: The desegregation of Little League baseball. *Journal of American Culture, 4,* 81–91.

Johnson, T. (1973). *My coach says . . . .* Williamsport, PA: Little League Baseball.

Joint Legislative Study Committee. (1976). *Joint legislative study on youth sports: Agency-sponsored sports—Phase I.* Lansing, MI: State of Michigan.

Joint Legislative Study Committee. (1978a). *Joint legislative study on youth sports: Agency-sponsored sports—Phase II*. Lansing, MI: State of Michigan.

Joint Legislative Study Committee. (1978b). *Joint legislative study on youth sports: Agency-sponsored sports—Phase III*. Lansing, MI: State of Michigan.

Kadjielski, M.A. (1977). As a flower needs sunshine: The origins of organized children's recreation in Philadelphia, 1886–1911. *Journal of Sport History, 4*, 169–188.

Lee, J. (1916). *Play in education*. New York: Scribner's.

Lewis, G. (1966). The Muscular Christianity movement. *Journal of Health, Physical Education and Recreation, 37*, 27–28, 42.

Lowman, C.L. (1947). The vulnerable age. *Journal of Health and Physical Education, 18*, 635.

Lucas, J.A. (1968). A prelude to the rise of sport: Ante-bellum America, 1850–1860. *Quest, 2*, 50–57.

Magill, R.A., Ash, M.J., & Smoll, F.L. (Eds.). (1978). *Children in sport: A contemporary anthology*. Champaign, IL: Human Kinetics.

Martens, R. (1978). *Joy and sadness in children's sports*. Champaign, IL: Human Kinetics.

Martens, R., Christina, R.W., Harvey, J.S., Jr., & Sharkey, B.J. (Eds.). (1981). *Coaching young athletes*. Champaign, IL: Human Kinetics.

Martens, R., & Seefeldt, V. (1979). *Guidelines for children's sports*. Washington, DC: American Alliance for Health, Physical Education, Recreation, and Dance.

Mergen, B. (1975). The discovery of children's play. *American Quarterly, 27*, 339–420.

Mitchell, E.D. (1932). Trends of athletes in junior high schools. *Journal of Health and Physical Education, 3*, 22.

Monroe, K. (1946). Hothouse for tennis champs. *Readers Digest, 49*, 22.

Moss, B., & Orion, W.H. (1939). The public school programs in health, physical education, and recreation. *Journal of Health and Physical Education, 10*, 435–439, 494.

National Collegiate Athletic Association. (1985). National youth sports program. *Brochure*. Mission, KS: Author.

National Council of Youth Sports Directors. (n.d.). *Brochure*.

National Recreation Congress. (1952). Are highly competitive sports desirable for juniors? *Recreation, 46*, 422–426.

National Youth Sport Coaching Association. (n.d.). *Brochure*. West Palm Beach, FL: Author.

Office of Youth Sports. (1979a). *Sportsline,* **1**(1), 2.

Office of Youth Sports. (1979b). *Sportsline,* **1**(2), 4.

Orlick, T., & Botterill, C. (1976). *Every kid can win.* Chicago: Nelson-Hall.

Paxton, H.T. (1949). Small boy's dreams come true. *Saturday Evening Post,* **221**, 26–27, 137–140.

Rader, B. (1983). *American sports: From the age of folk games to the age of spectators.* Englewood Cliffs, NJ: Prentice-Hall.

Rainwater, C.E. (1922). *The play movement in the United States: A study in community recreation.* Chicago: University of Chicago Press.

Ralbovsky, M. (1974). *Destiny's darlings.* New York: Hawthorne Books.

Reeve, A.B. (1910). The World's greatest athletic organization. *Outing,* **57**, 107–114.

Roberts, R. (1975, July). Strike out Little League. *Newsweek,* p. 11.

Rosen, A. (1967). *Baseball and your boy.* New York: Funk and Wagnall.

Seefeldt, V., Smoll, F.L., Smith, R.E., & Gould, D. (1981). *A winning philosophy for youth sports programs.* East Lansing, MI: Youth Sports Institute.

Smith, R.E., & Smoll, F.L. (1982a). *Leadership behaviors in youth sports: A theoretical model and research paradigm.* Unpublished manuscript.

Smith, R.E., & Smoll, F.L. (1982b). Psychological stress: A conceptual model and some intervention strategies in youth sports. In R.A. Magill, M.J. Ash, & F.L. Smoll (Eds.), *Children in sport: A contemporary anthology* (pp. 178–195). Champaign, IL: Human Kinetics.

Smith, R.E., Smoll, F.L., & Curtis, B. (1979). Coach effectiveness training: A cognitive behavioral approach to enhancing relationship skills in youth sport coaches. *Journal of Sport Psychology,* **1**, 59–78.

Smith, R.E., Smoll, F.L., & Hunt, E. (1977). A system for the behavioral assessment of athletic coaches. *Research Quarterly,* **48**, 401–407.

Smoll, F.L., & Smith, R.E. (1978). *Psychological perspectives in youth sports.* New York: Halsted Press.

Smoll, F.L., & Smith, R.E. (1979). *Improving relationship skills in youth sport coaches.* East Lansing, MI: Youth Sport Institute.

Smoll, F.L., & Smith, R.E. (1980). Psychologically oriented coach training programs: Design, implementation, and assessment. In C.H. Nadeau, W.R. Halliwell, K.M. Newell, & G.C. Roberts (Eds.), *Psychology of motor behavior and sport—1979* (pp. 112–129). Champaign, IL: Human Kinetics.

Special Olympics, Inc. (n.d.). *Special Olympics milestones.* Washington, DC: Author.

Tarkenton, F. (1970, October). Don't let your son play smallfry football. *Ladies Home Journal*, pp. 146–147.

Thomas, J. (Ed.). (1977). *Youth sports guide for coaches and parents*. Washington, DC: National Association for Sport and Physical Education.

Tutko, T., & Bruns, W. (1976). *Winning is everything and other American myths*. New York: Macmillan.

Underwood, J. (1975). Taking the fun out of games. *Sports Illustrated*, **43**, 86–98.

Voigt, D.Q. (1974). *A Little League journal*. Bowling Green, OH: Bowling Green University Press.

Wayman, F. (1950). Report of the president's committee on interschool competition in the elementary school. *Journal of Health, Physical Education, and Recreation*, **21**, 279–280, 313, 314.

Weiss, M.R., & Gould, D. (Eds.). (1986). *The 1984 Olympic Scientific Congress Proceedings: Vol 10. Sport for children and youths*. Champaign, IL: Human Kinetics.

Wingate, G.B. (1908). The public schools athletic league. *Outing*, **52**, 166.

# 2

# Gender Differences in Play Patterns and Sport Participation of North American Youth

**Crystal Fountain Branta**
**Mary Painter**
**Joy E. Kiger**

Sports and games are a genuine folk phenomenon in most societies and, as such, have revealed even subtle changes in a culture, its attitudes, or child behavior itself (Sutton-Smith & Rosenberg, 1961). Indicative of such cultural transformations are the profound changes found in the social roles of women during the past 40 years and their subsequent influence on the acceptance of the female in sports. Title IX and the inclusion of numerous new Olympic events for women are evidence of these changing attitudes on both the national and international levels. Girls have begun to play on ice hockey teams in recent years, and many American universities now offer touch football as an intramural sport for women. Surveys of the game and sport choices of children have indicated that, more than ever, girls are engaging in active sports and at earlier ages (Cratty, 1974; Fountain, 1978; Joint Legislative Study Committee, 1976). Will this earlier practice aid females in their subsequent sport performance? Only time will answer this question, but conceivably one reason the performance of males has been superior to that of females is that males have had more encouragement and opportunity to participate in sports at younger ages (Coakley, 1987).

Changing cultural norms are reflected in individual interests, lifestyles, and gender-role concepts. Traditionally, the female gender-role has been associated negatively with games, sports, and larger motor activities, whereas the male role has enjoyed a positive association (Fagot, 1978; Moss & Kagan, 1961). Environmental or social factors, rather than physical ones, have been more influential in determining masculinity and femininity (Tauber, 1979; Terman & Tyler, 1954). Coakley (1987) suggests that females have been less likely than males to receive encouragement for sport participation. Crum (1980) and Crum and Eckert (1985) found that the play of 8-year-old females stressed social interaction, cooperation, and individual performance, whereas that of males required high motor activity, physical skill, and direct competition. Lever (1976, 1978) indicated that boys played in larger groups and competed in more formal, complex games than girls. An examination, therefore, of gender differences in play activities and sports participation of children in our modern culture is appropriate, especially because social psychologists have long regarded play as an essential ingredient in preparing children for involvement in adult society (Stone, 1965). This review will focus on gender difference research in (a) physical and behavioral parameters of children, (b) characteristics of play behavior, and (c) trends in recreational sport participation.

## GENDER DIFFERENCES IN PHYSICAL AND BEHAVIORAL PARAMETERS OF CHILDREN

Indisputable differences on both physical and behavioral parameters exist between the means of the genders in our society. These differences could be the initial bases for the disparity in motor skill acquisition between males and females and, hence, in the success-to-failure ratio in sports for children of opposite genders. Because continued participation in an activity is directly related to the amount of success attained by the individual, recreational sport participation levels are probably highly diverse for girls and boys.

### Influences of Physical Differences

Structural discrepancies between females and males are numerous. Greater height and weight and a more massive skeleton are characteristic of the male.

In addition, the male has a larger muscle-to-fat ratio, a higher center of mass, greater proportional limb length, wider shoulders, and a more frontal insertion of the head of the femur into the pelvis than the female (Gray, 1973; Simmons, 1944; Tanner, 1962). In skill performance, these characteristics provide the average male with greater mechanical advantages, including a higher capacity for velocity and strength of motion and more efficiency in movements than the average female.

Performance of males and females on isolated motor skills has been documented previously (Branta, Haubenstricker, & Seefeldt, 1984). The results, in general, support the contention that there are gender differences in motor performances that may be partially attributable to physical or structural characteristics. Longitudinal data reported in that review show that the mean performance and relative change in scores favored males (ages 5 to 10 and 8 to 14 years) on the flexed-arm hang, horizontal jump, vertical jump, two agility runs, and the 30-yard dash. Females of the same ages scored higher on the sit-and-reach flexibility test. In fact, the flexibility of boys in that study decreased from ages 5 to 10 and 8 to 14 years. Children in the study were enrolled by their parents in an instructional program consisting of basic skills, sport skills, and swimming, and hence the typical gender disparity in encouragement, instruction, and practice would have been reduced.

In addition to structural parameters, physiological factors exist that vary by gender and usually afford an advantage in performance to the male. The absolute work capacity of the average male is approximately 20% greater than that of the typical female. Even when capacity is corrected for body size, performances remain at 15% in favor of the male. Oxygen consumption, vital capacity, blood volume, hemoglobin levels, cardiac output, and heart size per body mass are all lower in the female (Edington & Edgerton, 1976).

**Table 1**

**Percent of Participation in Selected Agency-Sponsored Sports**

| Sport | Male | Female |
|-------|------|--------|
| Baseball | 34.3 | 6.5 |
| Basketball | 17.4 | 10.0 |
| Tackle football | 12.7 | 2.4 |
| Wrestling | 6.8 | 2.0 |
| Swimming | 13.9 | 15.6 |
| Gymnastics | 4.9 | 9.6 |
| Figure skating | 2.0 | 4.6 |

*Note:*   Data collected from the *Joint Legislative Study Committee* (1976, pp. 63 and 77).

In general, these structural and physiological variances account for males excelling in sports requiring strength, endurance, power, and agility. Females are superior in movements that require balance and flexibility and also do well in sports where size and strength are not critical factors. Therefore, one would expect boys to participate more in sports such as tackle football, basketball, baseball, and wrestling and girls to be more involved in activities such as swimming, gymnastics, and figure skating. The youth sport study of the state of Michigan (Joint Legislative Study Committee, 1976) presented data that support these gender differences in degree of sport participation. Table 1 shows partial data of agency-sponsored participation as presented in this study. The percent involvement of males in the traditional male sports is much higher than that of females. Likewise, in the three sports more suited to the female constitution, the percentage of girls participating is higher than that of boys.

Data available on degree and type of involvement in recreational sports parallel that in agency-sponsored competition. Fountain (1978) and Seefeldt and Branta (1984) reported that males more often chose team games in their leisure time pursuits, whereas females participated most frequently in individual sports.

## Influence of Behavioral Differences

Gender differences in play behavior and sport participation cannot be attributed solely to derivatives of structural and physiological differences such as strength, power, and flexibility. Affective and cognitive dimensions are reflected in game and sport selection as well. Lever (1978) found that for 10- and 11-year-olds, boys' play was more complex than girls' on several factors, including interdependence among players, size of play group, and team formation. What behavioral differences exist between boys and girls that result in such characteristic differences in their play patterns?

Aggressive, independent behavior by males has been demonstrated in numerous studies of children (Crum, 1980; Goldberg & Lewis, 1969; Jacklin, Maccoby, & Dick, 1973; Maccoby, Doering, Jacklin, & Kraemer, 1981; Slovic, 1966; Spiro, 1956, 1958; Tauber, 1978; Whiting, 1963). In comparison to girls, boys exhibited greater willingness to take risks in games; demonstrated more active involvement in gross motor activities of an exploratory, vigorous nature; and showed less frustration and more active attempts to overcome barriers. Girls' behavior was directed toward sedentary, fine motor activites and was calmer and more regressive than the actions of boys. The play of girls tended to be more nurturant and self-grooming. Goldberg and Lewis (1969) recorded barrier frustration and crying in the female, as well as more dependence on and contact with the mother in a controlled play situation.

These male-female differences in play behavior occurred as early as 13 months of age and could possibly be related to a nuance in the mother-child relationship for a male versus that of a female child at 6 months of age (Goldberg

& Lewis, 1969; Kagan & Lewis, 1965). In these studies, mothers tended to allow males to cry longer in their cribs before comforting them and to cuddle the females more than their male children. Moreover, Fagot (1978) found that parents of 2-year-old children treated their toddlers differentially depending upon the children's gender. The parents reacted significantly more favorably to their offspring who were performing a same-sex-preferred behavior. In addition, these parents were more likely to react negatively to their daughters who were engaged in active, large motor activities and positively when the females exhibited adult-oriented, dependent behaviors. Coakley (1987) acknowledges this differential gender treatment that begins in the first 5 years of life.

Prenatal hormone levels also may affect human behavior according to gender. Ehrhardt and Baker (1981) found that females with adrenogenital syndrome (AGS), production of the male sex hormones prior to birth, were described as having high levels of intense physical energy when compared to their mothers and their unaffected female siblings. The AGS females showed a high degree of rough outdoor play over an extended period of time.

Moreover, the behavior of immature primates has been shown by several investigators to vary by gender as early as 2 months of age (Devore, 1965; Edington & Edgerton, 1976; Hamburg & Lunde, 1966; Harlow, 1962; Harlow & Lauersdorf, 1974). Infant male primates generally are rougher and more aggressive in play behavior and utilize large muscle groups in their activities; in contrast, young females tend to withdraw from rough contact play. These differences, like those for human children, seem to be related to early hormonal effects on the central nervous system (DeVore, 1965; Edington & Edgerton, 1976).

In addition to behavior variances, cognitive styles have been contrasted between the genders. Fourth-grade boys were guarded, evasive, and matter-of-fact in their cognition, limiting their responses to the task demands or rules. Cognitive styles of girls tended to be more imaginative, introspective, creative, and responsive to task changes (Minuchin, 1966).

From these data on typical gender differences in behavior and cognitive styles, certain predictions regarding sexually differential preferences in play patterns and sport involvement might be made. A greater participation of males in contact and high-risk sports is suggested, whereas greater female participation in individual, creative situations is expected. One confirmation of this prediction in competitive situations for children 5 to 16 years old is presented in Table 1. Additional support for this contention was supplied by Seefeldt and Branta (1984) in their historical review of recreational sport participation. In their comparative study, males demonstrated a much higher percentage of involvement in touch and tackle football and wrestling than females. Females had more play activities (e.g., playing jacks or jumping rope) that were not true sports than did males.

The differential preferences of boys and girls in their selection of play and sport activities do not reflect innate behavioral patterns in children. Many factors contribute to the gender-related choices in sport participation made by children.

Structural, physiological, cognitive, and socialization factors all play a role in gender differences that begin to appear in the informal play patterns of infants and preschool children and later in organized and recreational sport participation.

## GENDER-LINKED CHARACTERISTICS OF PLAY BEHAVIORS

Low-organization activities such as object manipulation, running, and chasing dominate the early years of the play lives of both boys and girls (Crosswell, 1898; Gross, 1976; Hurlock 1934/1971). From birth to age 3, play involves primarily sensory and motor exploration. Children constantly test their muscular control by practicing large, gross motor movements of their bodies and small, fine motor movements of objects. Motor development specialists have stated that basic locomotor patterns and eye-hand coordination are learned and perfected during ages 2 to 6 (Branta, Kiger, & Yager, 1985; Espenschade & Eckert, 1967).

During the preschool years (ages 3 to 6), symbolic play, imaginative play, and sociodramatic play take precedence over exploratory play for both genders (Gross, 1976; Hurlock, 1934/1971; Ulrich, 1968). Symbols are used for ideas about the world. These symbols may take the form of either concrete objects or roles assumed in dramatic play. Concerns of the real world via fantasy emerge. Ulrich (1968) states that these are the ages of imitation, drama, and experimentation with reality. The roles these young children assume and the symbols they utilize in their play, then, will probably influence the development of their motor skills and attitudes toward activity. These in turn might affect their subsequent sport participation, especially because during these years children seek a primary play group that will begin to develop rules for group behavior (Ulrich, 1968). By age 4, cooperative play is strong (Hurlock, 1934/1971), with the tendency to play in groups larger than two or three increasing across age (Parten, 1933/1971).

During the primary years (approximately ages 6 to 8), the emphasis in or characteristics of play change. Gender differentiation in play patterns becomes more readily apparent. According to Crum (1980), both 6-year-old girls and boys engage in closed activities with limited rules and only a few skills. They concentrate on individual performances, social interactions, and cooperation (e.g., taking turns). In general, both genders prefer same-sex play groups. Males, however, participate in cross-gender activities more often than females, suggesting that their view of gender-appropriate behavior is more flexible than that of females at age 6 (Crum, 1980; Crum & Eckert, 1985).

Over the years, females seem to become the more flexible gender in their views of gender-appropriate behavior. By age 8, males are responding to clear-cut role prescriptions in their preferences for mature, male-oriented activities, whereas females display greater role flexibility in their preferences for both male and female activities (Sutton-Smith, Rosenberg, & Morgan, 1963). Females overall still prefer small play groups composed of same-sex peers, have less structured activities with little participation in ball skills, and emphasize social conversation. The males, though, become involved with open skills using balls, activities requiring high motor skill ability, play groups of six or more, tasks requiring direct competition, and games with specific rules defining the outcome (Crum, 1980). Their play allows the opportunity for team membership and leadership practice, skills which may be beneficial in the adult professional life.

By age 10 the gender differences in play behavior appear to have become well established and are evidenced in the formal games of youth. Heavy involvement in sports by males 8 to 15 years old was originally documented by Lehman and Witty (1927). The list of games in which males participated consisted mostly of team sports, with baseball and football ranked first, second, or third throughout the age span. From ages 11 to 13, the composition of recreational sports for males changed, and by age 13 tennis began to rank within the top 10 activities.

The sport participation of females, taken from the same study, was low across the ages of 8 to 15 years. Roller skating was ranked within the top six activities by girls 8 to 13 years old, whereas basketball was an equally desirable choice for girls 11 to 15 years old. An item associated with sport, ''Doing Gymnasium Work,'' was ranked fifth or sixth on the list from ages 12 to 15 years. Although their sport participation was lower, the groups of girls from 14-1/2 to 18-1/2 years old were engaged in slightly more total activities than were males.

Support for the contention that girls are involved in more activities than boys was found at even younger ages by a more recent investigation (Sutton-Smith, Rosenberg, & Morgan, 1963). They reported that although play scale items were equally distributed between the genders at the third-grade level (approximately 8 years old), a sudden shift occurred at Grade 4 with more items differentiating girls from boys. Lehman and Witty (1927), in another research effort, had also shown participation curves for boys and girls to deviate most from 8-1/2 to 10-1/2 years of age for the entire range of play activities they investigated.

Even more recently, Lever (1976) reported marked gender differences between fifth graders and their play behaviors. Males played more competitive games than females, with 65% of the activities reported by males classified as formal games. Only 35% of the involvement of females was in such formal activities. Males participated in larger, more age-heterogeneous groups than females. Moreover, in groups of various aged children, young boys tried to play to the level of the older boys, whereas females tended to play to the level of the youngest participant. The games of males lasted longer than those of the females. Some suggested reasons for this time-in-play discrepancy include (a) the skill of males generally is higher than that of females so males are more challenged by the activity; (b) the lower motor skill of females does not keep the action exciting even when girls play games requiring a higher ceiling of skill; and (c) males resolve disputes quickly and continue with games, whereas females tend to break up the game when conflict arises thereby learning little about a judicial process.

Whereas gender differences in play and sport activities can be expected to appear and be at their strongest at 8 to 10 years, a decrease in participation for both boys and girls becomes evident sometime between 12 to 16 years. For both recreational activity (Eiferman, 1971) and agency competition (Joint Legislative Study Committee, 1976), the percentage of participants in competitive, rule-governed games was shown to increase up to age 11 to 12, followed by a decrease. This evidence supported the work by Lehman and Witty (1927) in which lower levels of sport involvement for both sexes were recorded at age 16. Ranks depicting males' sport involvement at age 16 evidenced a drastic drop to participation in only four sports ranked as follows: (a) basketball, (b) football, (c) baseball, and (d) tennis. Similarly, the ranks reflective of female sport participation in the same study indicated no major sport preferences at age 16.

The developmental nature of involvement in skilled pastimes and major sports has been documented by several investigators (Crosswell, 1898; Furfey, 1930; Hurlock, 1934/1971; Lehman & Witty, 1927; Sutton-Smith, 1959; Sutton-Smith & Rosenberg, 1961). After 8 years of age, children participate more in competitive play as organized athletics begin to predominate. Further verification of these data was found in an investigation of agency-sponsored competition (Joint Legislative Study Committee, 1976). These scientists found that the incidence of participation in most sports increased around 8 years of age for both genders. Games of skill increased in later youth, and play activity at adolescence was governed by strict rules and regulations in the form of games and athletic contests. Sutton-Smith (1959) stated that practically all play activity of children 11 years old or older was channeled into organized sports and that games of skill were played most by older children and males.

The middle years (approximately ages 7 to 12) become the "age of the club and team" (Gross, 1976, p. 15). Participation in the skills and games of the culture is important to young people of this age. The emphasis is on precision and rule following. These findings imply that learning and development of the motor skills must be prerequisite to participation in the desirable peer activities. The critical questions to be asked are, What happens between 6 and 8 years to cause the change in play, particularly of males? and, How could this transition be facilitated in females so that more females might also benefit from experiences in team membership and leadership skills in recreational sports?

## GENDER-RELATED TRENDS
## IN RECREATIONAL SPORT PARTICIPATION

Fountain (1978) examined the participation of almost 90,000 Michigan children in 35 recreational sports and found boys and girls to be active in a variety of sports during their school-age years. Children aged 5 to 16 were asked to rate the degree of their involvement in selected sports by responding "often," "sometimes," or "never." From their responses, Fountain was able to examine popularity trends in sport participation, categorize sports on the basis of gender involvement, and classify sports with regard to pattern of participation at various ages. The material that follows reflects results obtained in that study.

## Popularity Trends of Selected Sports

Within the 20 most popular sports for each sex, 18 of them were common to both genders (see Table 2). In fact, 5 sports (bicycling, swimming, basketball, softball, and kickball) were common to both genders within the top 10-ranked sports. Moreover, similarities between males and females were seen in the bottom 4 rankings. Karate, judo, cross-country skiing, and scuba diving ranked last for both boys and girls, and never more than a 6% between-gender difference existed in the levels of participation for any one of these activities.

Although both males and females marked 12 individual/dual sports in the 20 most popular ones, the distribution of those activities varied. Only 4 of the 12 individual/dual sports were ranked in the top 10 by males, whereas females ranked 6 of the 12 in the top 10. Girls participated most frequently in individual/dual activities, whereas boys were involved most in team games.

Bicycling ranked as the most popular activity with 94% involvement by males and 95% by females. Swimming ranked second with 89% and 90% participation, respectively. Basketball for males was the only other activity showing participation greater than 80%. A striking occurrence in this investigation, however, was that well over half of the sample indicated participation in the top 10 sports. In fact, boys had a total of 17 sports in which at least 50% participated, and girls had 13 such sports. Although these percentages of participation were quite high, the levels for females dropped more rapidly than those of the males. Participation for males showed 26 sports with levels of 30% or more, whereas female participation exceeded 30% in only 21 sports.

When considering just those subjects who participated "often" as compared to "total" participation (sum of those who participated "often" and "sometimes"), levels of involvement in recreational sport were still quite high. At least one third of the sample engaged in 10 sports for males and 7 for females. The levels of involvement were similar for boys and girls, especially within the highest and lowest ranked activities. Also, as in the figures for "total" participation, the percent of females involved "often" in activities decreased more rapidly as one descended the ranks than the percents for males.

The "total" percentage of participation by females in sports typically considered masculine was found to be extensive (baseball, 45%; touch football, 40%; tackle football, 32%). Even within the lowest ranked sports in the column for females, wrestling was marked by 20% of the respondents and weight lifting by 14%. In addition, ice hockey was played by 9% of the girls. These figures,

**Table 2**

**Most Popular Sports Ranked by Total Percent of Participation, Independent of Age From 5–16 Years**

| | Male | | | Female | |
|---|---|---|---|---|---|
| Rank | Sport | Percent | Rank | Sport | Percent |
| 1 | Bicycling[a] | 94 | 1 | Bicycling[a] | 95 |
| 2 | Swimming[a] | 89 | 2 | Swimming[a] | 90 |
| 3 | Basketball[a] | 82 | 3 | Softball[a] | 73 |
| 4 | Softball[a] | 79 | 4 | Roller skating[a] | 73 |
| 5 | Tackle football[a] | 74 | 5 | Kickball[a] | 72 |
| 6 | Baseball[a] | 73 | 6 | Ice skating[a] | 66 |
| 7 | Touch football[a] | 69 | 6 | Basketball[a] | 66 |
| 7 | Kickball[a] | 69 | 8 | Gymnastics[a] | 61 |
| 9 | Table tennis[a] | 65 | 9 | Volleyball[a] | 60 |
| 10 | Bowling[a] | 64 | 10 | Badminton[a] | 58 |
| 11 | Ice skating[a] | 62 | 10 | Table tennis[a] | 58 |
| 12 | Roller skating[a] | 58 | 12 | Bowling[a] | 57 |
| 12 | Jogging[a] | 58 | 13 | Jogging[a] | 54 |
| 14 | Wrestling | 55 | 14 | Tennis[a] | 48 |
| 14 | Volleyball[a] | 55 | 15 | Baseball[a] | 45 |
| 16 | Badminton[a] | 54 | 16 | Horseback riding | 44 |
| 17 | Weight lifting | 51 | 17 | Touch football[a] | 40 |
| 18 | Tennis[a] | 48 | 18 | Soccer[a] | 37 |
| 19 | Soccer[a] | 47 | 19 | Tackle football[a] | 32 |
| 20 | Gymnastics | 40 | 19 | Miniature golf | 32 |
| 21 | Miniature golf | 39 | 21 | Track & field | 30 |
| 21 | Track & field | 39 | 22 | Wrestling | 20 |
| 23 | Floor hockey | 38 | 23 | Floor hockey | 19 |
| 24 | Horseback riding | 35 | 24 | Water skiing | 17 |
| 25 | Archery | 32 | 25 | Synchronized swimming | 14 |
| 25 | Ice hockey | 32 | 25 | Weight lifting | 14 |
| 27 | Golf | 25 | 27 | Archery | 13 |
| 28 | Snorkeling | 22 | 28 | Downhill skiing | 12 |
| 29 | Water skiing | 21 | 29 | Golf | 10 |
| 30 | Downhill skiing | 14 | 30 | Ice hockey | 9 |
| 31 | Synchronized swimming | 12 | 31 | Snorkeling | 8 |
| 32 | Karate | 11 | 32 | Karate | 5 |
| 33 | Judo | 7 | 32 | Cross-country skiing | 5 |
| 34 | Cross-country skiing | 6 | 34 | Judo | 3 |
| 35 | Scuba diving | 5 | 35 | Scuba diving | 2 |

[a]Top 20 sports rated by both genders as most popular.

however, summarize all females indicating participation in these sports. When only the "often" responses of female participation were considered, none of the typically masculine sports had levels higher than 16% (baseball, 16%; touch football, 11%; tackle football, 9%; wrestling, 7%; ice hockey, 2%; and weight lifting, 2%).

## Categorization of Sports on the Basis of Gender

Because the data on the extent of involvement revealed some differences between the genders in amount of "often" participation and the choices of midranked activities, Fountain (1978) categorized sports into those that were predominantly male or female. Because of the extremely large sample size (approximately 90,000), any sport with differences greater than 1% in participation between males and females could have been shown to be statistically significant. These differences, however, are probably trivial and would not be meaningful to people who coordinate or teach physical activities and/or regulate the planning of facilities. Therefore, differences in participation between males and females of 15% were deemed significant. Those sports differentiating between males and females on this basis are listed in Table 3.

**Table 3**

**Sports Differentiating Between Genders (Differences in "Total" Percent Participation are ≥ 15%)**

| Male | Female |
| --- | --- |
| Archery | Gymnastics |
| Baseball[a] | Roller skating |
| Basketball[a] | |
| Tackle football[a] | |
| Touch football[a] | |
| Golf | |
| Floor hockey | |
| Ice hockey | |
| Weight lifting[a] | |
| Wrestling[a] | |

[a]Participation on "often" basis ≥ 15%.

Males had 10 sports in which their total levels of participation exceeded that of the females by at least 15%. In contrast, females had only gymnastics and roller skating in which their participation exceeded that of males by the same level. Again, if one considers only the respondents who participated ''often'' in activities as opposed to ''total'' involvement, the male column contained six sports (baseball, basketball, tackle football, touch football, weight lifting, and wrestling), whereas females did not exceed the involvement of males by 15% or more in any activity.

### Categorization of Sports on the Basis of Participation Pattern

When examining participation in recreational sports across the ages of 5 to 16 years, several trends in the data emerged (Fountain, 1978). Sports could be classified into three categories of participant involvement: (a) those that increased with chronological age, peaked at a certain age, and then leveled off; (b) those that increased with chronological age, peaked, and then declined; or (c) those that increased throughout the age range.

The most common trend by age, regardless of gender, was for sport participation to increase, peak at age 12 to 13, and then remain constant until 16 years (see Table 4). Of the 70 sports (35 sports × 2 genders) investigated, 38 fell into this category. Sports in which participation levels increased with chronological age, peaked, and then declined, designated the second classification of sports by age (see Table 5). Twenty-four of the 70 possible activities were included in this category. The third classification includes sports in which participation increased throughout ages 5 to 16 (see Table 6). All sports in this category began

### Table 4

**Sports With Participation That Increased, Peaked, Then Leveled Throughout Ages 5–16 for Both Genders**

| | |
|---|---|
| Archery | Karate |
| Badminton | Scuba diving |
| Bicycling | Cross-country skiing |
| Bowling | Snorkeling |
| Touch football | Swimming |
| Golf (females) | Synchronized swimming |
| Miniature golf | Table tennis (females) |
| Horseback riding | Tennis (females) |
| Ice hockey | Volleyball |
| Jogging | Weight lifting (females) |
| Judo | |

**Table 5**

**Sports With Participation That Increased, Peaked, Then Declined Throughout Ages 5–16 for Both Genders**

| | |
|---|---|
| Baseball | Kickball |
| Softball | Ice skating |
| Basketball | Roller skating |
| Tackle football | Soccer |
| Gymnastics | Track & field |
| Floor hockey | Wrestling |

**Table 6**

**Sports With Participation That Increased Throughout Ages 5–16 Years for Both Genders**

| | |
|---|---|
| Downhill skiing | Table tennis (males) |
| Water skiing | Tennis (males) |
| Golf (males) | Weight lifting (males) |

with low levels of involvement at ages 5 to 7, and participation continually increased through age 16.

In golf, table tennis, tennis, and weight lifting, patterns of participation by age were dissimilar for males and females. In these four sports, participation for males continued to increase through age 16 (see Table 6), whereas that for females peaked and then leveled (see Table 4). Another common characteristic was for the percentage of "often" participation to approach or exceed that of "sometimes," especially for the four sports of golf, table tennis, tennis, and weight lifting for males only. This factor is interesting in that the usual pattern of participation in this study was for "sometimes" involvement to be higher than that for "often." For females the amount of participation "sometimes" remained higher throughout all ages than for "often."

Young people aged 5 to 16 participate extensively in recreational sports. The type of sports in which males and females indicate involvement is quite similar, with males choosing slightly more team games than females. In addition, the patterns of participation across age are virtually the same when examined by gender. Therefore, directors of sport programs should modify or expand the offerings of activities, equipment, facilities, and instruction to account for the high interest and amounts of participation in recreational sports. Other implications relating to program design are to allow males a few more choices of team games and to incorporate more individual/dual activities into the curricula for females.

Although males had more sports in which their participation levels were at least 15% greater than that for females, young women showed considerable involvement in sports typically considered masculine. Rules and equipment should be carefully examined and possibly adapted for the safety of those females who wish to participate in contact sports. For example, flag football could be provided for school-aged girls as it now is for women in many American universities. Further study is needed to determine how, if at all, contact sports should be modified for participation by females, or indeed if females should be encouraged to participate in such sports. In addition, some semicontact team sports (e.g., soccer, basketball) show high popularity for each gender, require a small amount of equipment, and offer a good activity for increased fitness levels of youth. These types of sports should be considered for inclusion when developing curricula and should be reviewed for possible incorporation as coeducational pursuits.

## SUMMARY

Several factors that may influence differences in play activities and sport participation patterns of males and females have been discussed. Physical and behavioral parameters were noted, and implications for effects on sport involvement were provided. Generally, the structural and physiological factors that differ between the genders account for males excelling in sports requiring power, strength, and agility, whereas females are better in balance and flexibility movements. Research has shown that males participate more in rough activities and contact sports, whereas females prefer quieter activities and individual sports.

Behavioral and cognitive styles vary by gender. Males show and are rewarded for aggressive, independent behavior and are more willing to take risks. Females are calmer and more regressive but creative; the parents of young girls react positively to these behaviors.

The developmental nature of involvement in play and major sports was discussed. Low organization activities at early ages have been shown to give way to competitive athletics around 8 years of age, with an emphasis on precision and rule following. This athletic involvement peaks during the middle years (ages 7 to 12). Marked gender differences in play behaviors occur during these years.

Data from a study of about 90,000 Michigan youth were presented. The results suggest that for most of the recreational sports in which total levels of participation were high, a trend of moderate to high amounts of involvement at the early ages of 5 to 7 is present. Participation at younger ages might influence the extent to which individuals become involved in sports at later ages. Males had somewhat higher percents of involvement throughout most sports, maintained these levels longer, and had relatively higher degrees of "often" involvement than did females. Sports were grouped into three distinct categories according to patterns of participation across the ages of 5 to 16. Trends for both genders in the three categories are remarkably similar.

## REFERENCES

Branta, C., Haubenstricker, J., & Seefeldt, V. (1984). Age changes in motor skills during childhood and adolescence. In R.L. Terjung (Ed.), *Exercise and sport sciences reviews* (pp. 467–520). Lexington, MA: The Collamore Press.

Branta, C.F., Kiger, J., & Yager, M. (1985, April). *Profiles of the motor performance of pre-school age children*. Paper presented at the meeting of the American Alliance for Health, Physical Education, Recreation, and Dance, Atlanta, GA.

Coakley, J. (1987). Children and the sport socialization process. In D. Gould & M. Weiss (Eds.), *Advances in pediatric sport sciences: Vol 2. Behavioral Issues* (pp. 43–60). Champaign, IL: Human Kinetics.

Cratty, B.J. (1974). *Children and youth in competitive sport*. Freeport, NY: Educational Activities.

Crosswell, T.R. (1898). Amusements of Worchester school children. *The Pedagogical Seminary, 6*, 314–371.

Crum, J.F. (1980). *An observational study of the play patterns of elementary school children*. Unpublished doctoral dissertation, University of California, Berkeley.

Crum, J.F., & Eckert, H.M. (1985). Play patterns of primary school children. In J.E. Clark & J.H. Humphrey (Eds.), *Motor development: Current selected research* (Vol. 1, pp. 99–114). Princeton, NJ: Princeton Book Company.

DeVore, I. (1965). *Primate behavior*. New York: Holt, Rinehart, and Winston.

Edington, D.W., & Edgerton, V.T. (1976). *The biology of physical activity*. Boston: Houghton-Mifflin.

Ehrhardt, A.A., & Baker, S.W. (1981). Fetal androgens, human central nervous system differentiation, and behavioral sex differences. In E.M. Hetherington & R.D. Parke (Eds.), *Contemporary readings in child psychology* (2nd ed., pp. 380–389). New York: McGraw-Hill.

Eiferman, R.R. (1971). Social play in childhood. In R.E. Herron & B. Sutton-Smith (Eds.), *Child's play*, (pp. 270–297). New York: John Wiley.

Espenschade, A.S., & Eckert, H.M. (1967). *Motor development*. Columbus, OH: Charles E. Merrill.

Fagot, B.I. (1978). The influence of sex of child on parental reactions to children. *Child Development, 42*(2), 459–465.

Fountain, C.D. (1978). *Sex and age differences in the recreational sport participation of children*. Unpublished master's thesis, Michigan State University, East Lansing.

Furfey, P.H. (1930). *The growing boy*. New York: Macmillan.

Goldberg, S., & Lewis, M. (1969). Play behavior in the year old infant: Early sex differences. *Child Development, 40*, 21–31.

Gray, H. (1973). *Anatomy of the human body* (29th ed.). Philadelphia: Lea & Febiger.

Gross, D.W. (1976). Play and thinking. In P.M. Markun (Ed.), *Play: Children's business* (pp. 11–16). Washington, DC: Association for Childhood Educational International.

Hamburg, D.A., & Lunde, D.I. (1966). Sex hormones in the development of sex differences in human behavior. In E.E. Maccoby (Ed.), *The development of sex differences* (pp. 1–24). Stanford, CA: Stanford University Press.

Harlow, H. (1962). The heterosexual affection system in monkeys. *American Psychologist, 17*, 1–9.

Harlow, H.F., & Lauersdorf, H.E. (1974). Sex differences in passion and play. *Perspectives in Biology and Medicine, 17*, 348–360.

Hurlock, E.B. (1971). Experimental investigations of childhood play. In R.E. Herron & B. Sutton-Smith (Eds.), *Child's play* (pp. 51–70). New York: John Wiley & Sons. (Reprinted from *Psychological Bulletin*, 1934, *31*, 47–66)

Jacklin, C.N., Maccoby, E.E., & Dick, A.E. (1973). Barrier behavior and toy preference: Sex differences (and their absence) in the year-old child. *Child Development, 44*, 196–200.

Joint Legislative Study Committee. (1976). *Joint legislative study on youth sports programs*. Lansing, MI: State of Michigan.

Kagan, J., & Lewis, M. (1965). Studies of attention in the human infant. *Merrill-Palmer Quarterly, 11*, 95–127.

Lehman, H.C., & Witty, P.A. (1927). *The psychology of play activities*. New York: Barnes.

Lever, J. (1976). Sex differences in the games children play. *Social Problems, 23*, 478–487.

Lever, J. (1978). Sex differences in the complexity of children's play and games. *American Sociological Review, 43*, 471–483.

Maccoby, E.E., Doering, C.H., Jacklin, C.N., & Kraemer, H. (1981). Concentrations of sex hormones in umbilical cord blood: Their relation to sex and birth order of infants. In E.M. Hetherington & R.D. Parke (Eds.), *Contempory readings in child psychology* (pp. 220–226). New York: McGraw-Hill.

Minuchin, P. (1966). Sex differences in children: Research findings in an educational context. *The National Elementary Principal, 46*, 45–48.

Moss, H.A., & Kagan, J. (1961). Stability of achievement and recognition seeking behavior from early childhood through adulthood. *Journal of Abnormal Psychology, 62*, 504–513.

Parten, M.B. (1971). Social play among preschool children. In R.E. Herron & B. Sutton-Smith (Eds.), *Child's play* (pp. 83–95). New York: John Wiley & Sons. (Reprinted from *Journal of Abnormal and Social Psychology*, 1933, 28, 136–147)

Seefeldt, V., & Branta, C.F. (1984). Patterns of participation in children's sports. In J.R. Thomas (Ed.), *Motor development during childhood and adolescence* (pp. 190–211). Minneapolis: Burgess.

Simmons, K. (1944). Physical growth and development. *Monograph of the Society for Research in Child Development, 9* (1, Serial No. 37).

Slovic, L. (1966). Risk-taking in children: Age and sex differences. *Child Development, 37*, 169–176.

Spiro, M.E. (1956). *Kibbutz: Venture in utopia*. Cambridge: Harvard University Press.

Spiro, M.E. (1958). *Children of the kibbutz*. Cambridge: Harvard University Press.

Stone, G.P. (1965). The play of little children. *Quest, 4*, 23–31.

Sutton-Smith, B. (1959). *The games of New Zealand children*. Berkeley: University of California Press.

Sutton-Smith, B., & Rosenberg, B.G. (1961). Sixty years of historical change in the game preferences of American children. *Journal of American Folklore, 74*, 17–46.

Sutton-Smith, B., Rosenberg, B.G., & Morgan, E.F., Jr. (1963). Development of sex differences in play choices during preadolescence. *Child Development, 34*, 119–126.

Tanner, J.M. (1962). *Growth at adolescence*. Oxford: Blackwell Scientific.

Tauber, M.A. (1979). Parental socialization techniques and sex differences in children's play. *Child Development, 50*, 225–234.

Terman, L., & Tyler, L.E. (1954). Psychological sex differences. In L. Carmichael (Ed.), *Manual of child psychology* (pp. 1064–1114). New York: Wiley.

Ulrich, C. (1968). *The social matrix of physical education*. Englewood Cliffs, NJ: Prentice-Hall.

Whiting, B.B. (Ed.). (1963). *Six cultures: Studies of child rearing*. New York: John Wiley & Sons.

# 3

# Children and the Sport Socialization Process

**Jay J. Coakley**

What leads children to become involved in sports, especially organized sports? What happens to children as a result of their participation? And what are children looking for in their sport experiences? Although social scientists do not have definitive answers to these three questions, we know enough to help people understand some of what goes on in the sport socialization process.

Before dealing with these questions, we must identify whom and what we will be discussing in this chapter. First, when we refer to children we are talking about young people under 13 years old. Second, the term *sports* will be used in two ways. *Informal sports* will refer to the pickup games played by children, games that they organize and control themselves. *Organized youth sports* will refer to adult-controlled sport programs, programs in which there are formally organized teams and leagues with coaches and schedules. Third, the term *socialization* will be used to refer to the process of social interaction through which people develop, extend, and change their ideas about who they are and how they relate to the world around them. Socialization is a never-ending process; as long as social interaction occurs, our ideas about ourselves are subject to growth and change.

## SOCIALIZATION INTO SPORTS

Suprisingly, little research prevails on what leads children to begin and continue their involvement in sports. With the widespread media coverage of sports since the early 1960s, we know that most children become familiar with organized, competitive games before they enter elementary school. Many parents encourage their children, especially their sons, to identify with popular professional athletes in sports receiving heavy media attention. To the extent that parents value and give their attention to sports, children learn to see sports as worthwhile activities. Furthermore, the first experiences that young children have with sport activities generally occur within the context of the family (Berlage, 1982). Parents may give them sport equipment and sport clothing as presents; parents may play catch with them, take them skating or swimming, or show them how to bounce a basketball; and parents may explain to them what is involved in running a race, competing for rewards, and achieving personal goals. Of course, not all families are the same, nor are all children in any one family treated the same way.

### Family Income, Single Parents, and Socialization Into Sports

Children in low-income or single-parent families do not usually have the same opportunities as other children when it comes to being socialized into sports. Growing up poor usually means that sports equipment is scarce and that exposure to different kinds of sports is very limited. In general, family resources influence the type and number of sports to which children are introduced early in their lives. Furthermore, research suggests that parental expectations about the socialization outcomes of youth sport participation vary with the socioeconomic status of families (Watson, 1977). For example, working-class parents often view participation as an opportunity for their children to learn how to respond to authority figures and to conform to the expectations of others in competitive settings. Middle-class parents, on the other hand, often view participation as an opportunity for their children to learn game skills along with self-directed behaviors in environments requiring teamwork and cooperation. More research is needed on this issue, but patterns of socialization into sports are likely influenced by parental expectations associated with the sport experience, and parental expectations vary with socioeconomic factors such as their incomes, occupations, and educational backgrounds.

Children with single parents may also have limited exposure to sport activities early in their lives. Although no research exists on this topic, single parents, especially mothers, might not have the financial resources, the time, or the experiences enabling them to personally encourage their children to become involved in sports. Single mothers may not feel comfortable teaching their children how to throw a ball or how to do other things they themselves never learned to do when they were younger. If a single mother must work long hours to support her children, she is not likely to have the money or the time to buy equipment or supervise the learning of sport skills. Research is needed on this topic to see if children in single-parent families have different sport participation patterns than other children as they get older. At this time, we can only make some educated guesses.

## Race and Socialization Into Sports

Although separating the effects of race and socioeconomic status is difficult, evidence suggests that at least some black children, especially males with above-average athletic skills, are socialized into sports through different forms of encouragement than is received by their white counterparts (Braddock, 1980; Oliver, 1980). Despite the misleading and mythical nature of the belief that sport offers blacks more opportunities than other occupational spheres in American society, many black children are encouraged to view sport as a means for upward social mobility. This encouragement gets stronger as they move through adolescence and begin to perceive barriers to success in fields outside of sport and entertainment (Harris & Hunt, 1984).

Although the family exerts an important influence on the way black children are introduced to sport, sources of support outside the family are also important. Encouragement from same-sex peers, teachers, coaches, and the community in general may be more influential for blacks than for whites. But whether this is due to race-related or class-related factors is not known. Also, in some black communities physical movement may be defined in different ways than it is in white communities. If movement among black children is associated with expressive meanings and if movement has important social implications that do not exist among many white children, the dynamics of socialization into sport would be quite different for the two races. At this point we know little about this issue; research is needed.

## Gender and Socialization Into Sports

Within families, boys and girls are often introduced to physical activities and sports differently. As infants, girls are handled more gently and protectively than boys, and they are watched over more closely before and after they begin to walk. Boys, on the other hand, are thrown into the air more often, given more toys requiring active play and the use of motor skills, and allowed to explore more of their physical environments without parental supervision and assistance

(Lewis, 1972a, 1972b). This pattern of protecting (and constraining) girls and encouraging the physical independence of boys is usually maintained through childhood (Caplan, 1981; Chafetz, 1978; Coakley, 1986b; Langlois & Downs, 1980).

Between the ages of 2 and 5, children identify themselves as either male or female and begin to form ideas about what is expected from members of each sex. Although individual ideas differ by social class and family, general patterns of expectations exist in Western culture. In most North American families, for example, young girls are not discouraged from playing sports, but they are usually socialized differently than their brothers in at least two respects. First, they are less likely to learn that physical activities and achievements in sports can or should be uniquely important sources of rewards in their lives. Second, their play time is more likely to be regulated and controlled by their parents. For example, when a 10-year-old girl asks one of her parents for permission to play, she may hear something like this: "I think it is great that you're going to play; you have my permission *as long as* you

- stay in the house";
- stay close to the house";
- go with a friend";
- play with children whom I know";
- don't do anything dangerous";
- keep your clothes clean";
- don't play rough or get hurt";
- don't get into fights or arguments with your friends";
- watch your little brother";
- get home at exactly 4 o'clock—no later!"; or
- set the table in time for dinner."

This form of "conditional permission" not only influences the skill development of little girls, but it constrains the nature of the games and informal sports they play with their friends as they get older. They focus on activities with a "best friend" and they are less likely to play complex, competitive games in large groups of age-mixed participants (Lever, 1976, 1978).

Boys have fewer parental constraints and usually move beyond their sisters in the development of physical skills at rather young ages. As they get older they are more confident when it comes to taking advantage of opportunities to participate in both informal sports and organized sport programs. As girls enter school they are less likely than their male counterparts to receive strong support from family, peers, teachers, coaches, and the general community to begin and continue their involvement in sports. For boys, sport participation is seen as being directly linked to their development as men. For girls, sport participation is seldom linked to becoming a woman. Such issues become crucial as adolescence is approached.

**General Research Findings on Socialization Into Sports**

Unfortunately, most of the information we have about socialization into sports comes from studies of white, male high school and college athletes or top-level amateurs. In these studies the subjects have usually been asked to recall the special people who influenced their decisions to participate in sport at particular times while they were growing up. Occasionally, information from elite athletes has been compared to information from others, but the use of comparison groups has been rare. Therefore, we know little about those who never maintained active participation beyond early adolescence or about those who confined their participation to informal games or recreational programs.

However, on a general level we do know that a child's initial involvement in either informal or organized sports is influenced by (a) the availability of opportunities; (b) support from family members, peers, role models, and the general community; and (c) the child's self-perception as a potential participant. Research is especially needed on this third factor. Knowledge about how a child's decision to participate in sports is tied to identity, body image, self-esteem, and experiences in physical activities during early childhood would be helpful, as would information about how sport participation is incorporated into children's everyday life events and self-conceptions. Becoming involved in sports means different things to different children. Adults, including parents and coaches, need to be sensitive to the individual meanings assigned to sport experiences. Knowing why children are involved enables us to help them grow in positive directions from their sport experiences. This brings us to our next topic: What happens to children who participate in sports?

## THE CONSEQUENCES OF SPORT PARTICIPATION AMONG CHILDREN

When parents encourage their children to participate in sports, they assume that the consequences of participation will be positive. However, research on this issue has produced little evidence that would lead to this conclusion. The notion that participation in organized sport programs produces good citizens, moral development, or other traits generally associated with good character receives no consistent support (Coakley, 1986a; Coakley & Bredemeier, 1985;

Kleiber & Kelly, 1980; Loy, McPherson, & Kenyon, 1978; McPherson, 1985). This does not mean that good things do not happen to the participants in these programs. They do happen, but they are probably less frequent and less dramatic than many people believe.

The mistaken belief that participation in sport automatically leads to the development of good character is grounded in three factors. First, organized sport programs tend to attract participants with certain characteristics. For example, children with low self-confidence and poorly developed physical skills are less likely to try out for and make organized teams than children who are confident and highly skilled (McGuire & Cook, 1983; Medrich, Roizen, Rubin, & Buckley, 1982; Orlick & Botterill, 1975; Roberts, Kleiber, & Duda, 1981). Furthermore, those with traits defined as undesirable by coaches may be cut from teams or discouraged from continuing their participation. This means that many of the participants in organized programs are those who already measure high on what people would describe as good character. They are selected into sport programs and then use those programs as settings to display and nurture their attributes.

A second reason that people believe sport builds character is that they usually focus much of their attention on the most outstanding young people in organized programs. They not only assume that those young people had their characters built in sport but also that if the characters of some children are built in sport, all other children must be experiencing the same consequences. Research shows that these assumptions are generally inaccurate.

A third reason for believing that sport builds character is that athletes have opportunities to demonstrate their skills publicly. Athletes at any level of competition often face challenging situations in which their behaviors are visible and easily evaluated. Because the everyday life activities of adults and children rarely overlap in most industrial societies, most adults seldom have opportunities to see children in such challenging situations. When children demonstrate their abilities in sports, the adults watching them often conclude that those abilities were created through sport participation. However, what probably happens is that sport gives adults, especially parents, a chance to see children display previously unseen skills and attributes that have already been acquired during the normal processes of growth and maturation.

Although research has not shown that sport participation systematically produces positive socialization outcomes, it suggests that when good outcomes do occur they are tied to the social relationships occasioned by sport involvement. The physical experience of sport participation by itself does little. Getting hits and scoring goals are not nearly as important as the feedback children receive from those who are important people in their lives. Adults and peers mediate sport experiences for children. The experiences take on meaning for children through their relationships with others. And through those relationships definitions of success and failure are developed and applied to what happens on the playing fields.

Unfortunately, most research on the consequences of participation has been designed so that those involved in sports have simply been compared with those who are not involved. This means that even when researchers have found differences between these two groups, they could not conclude that the differences were caused by sport participation. Even if the differences were caused by participation, nothing could be said about what aspects of the overall sport experience produced the differences. The consequences of being involved in sports are thus very difficult to pinpoint. However, we do know some things that are useful in understanding what happens and what doesn't happen to children in sport. The following sections will at least partially address five important issues about the consequences of participation.

## Organized Sport Programs' Effect on Parent-Child Relationships

The *informal* games of children do not usually influence family life. Children get together on their own and use makeshift equipment and unofficial playing fields. They have no uniforms, lineups, scoreboards, or after-game treats. But the practices and games in *organized* sport programs are different. A family commitment of time, money, and personal involvement is often demanded when children participate in these programs. Parents may have to adjust meal schedules, weekend activities, work routines, and vacation times to get their children to practices and games and to watch them compete (Berlage, 1982; Snyder & Purdy, 1982).

Ash (1978) has suggested that organized sport programs for children have had "as much of an impact on family structure and behavior as any other societal event" since the 1950s (p. 176). In support of this rather strong statement, national survey data show that 80% of parents with children participating in these programs attend games on a frequent basis (*Miller Lite Report*, 1983). Of course, family involvement does not automatically lead to positive changes in the nature of family relationships. But during a time when so many activities in industrial societies are age-segregated, these programs provide settings within which parents and children can interact with one another.

However, we must be careful not to jump to the conclusion that good things always happen whenever parents and children get together. Studies have shown that parental involvement in organized sport programs can negatively affect family relationships and the psychological well-being of their children (State of Michigan, 1978; Yablonsky & Brower, 1979). Unlike many other activities involving both parents and children, sports have the potential for producing negative emotions and negative feedback in family relationships. The most potentially destructive situation occurs when children believe that their relationships with one or both parents depend on continued involvement in sport or on the quality of their athletic performances.

To avoid this problem, parents must be aware of the differences between pressure and encouragement in their children's minds. Without making a constant supportive effort to understand how children perceive parental feedback, parents may unwittingly put destructive pressure on their children. To illustrate how this might happen, put yourself in the shoes ($80 top-of-the-line athletic shoes) of an 11-year-old in a sport program. As an 11-year-old you clearly remember that things were different at home before you started playing organized sports. In the past, your parents always let you know how hard they worked for the $3 they gave you for a movie. In fact, they often gave lectures on how money did not grow on trees. But now that you are an athlete, they do not hesitate to spend significant amounts of money every season to outfit you in high-quality sports gear and to pay for entry and instructional fees. After years of hearing how busy your parents were and how they needed a vacation, they are now giving up their weekends to drive you to games, meets, and practices. They even changed the family vacation to enable the whole family to attend your playoffs. They fix special dinners five nights a week so you can get to practice on time. They try to come home from work early so they can see part of your practices, and they tell you how proud they are of you because of your involvement. At the same time they could not make it to the quarterly PTA meeting at which your latest art project was displayed, and they complained about how difficult it was for them to fit a parent-teacher conference into their busy schedules even though your academic progress at school was going to be discussed. Of course, they continued to tell you how important school was and that sport was just for fun. But their behavior told you otherwise.

Under these conditions, most 11-year-olds would conclude that their sport involvement is much more important than their parents say it is. If parents are not careful about the content of these unspoken messages, they can lead their children to think that being an athlete is a prerequisite for continued parental interest and concern. Such a thought constitutes pressure, not encouragement. More research is needed on this topic, but at least one study has documented parents as a possible source of pressure in young athletes' lives (Scanlon & Lewthwaite, 1984).

In summary, whether the participation of children in organized sport programs has any systematic effect on family relationships is not known. Participation has sometimes brought families together, caused problems, or simply provided settings for family members to play out their relationships with one another in the same ways they would in other settings. Research is needed to discover the conditions under which each of these consequences occurs. In the meantime, parents must be aware of all the positive and negative things that could be happening with family relationships when a child is involved in sports.

## Organized Sport Programs' Influence on Children's Abilities to Create and Maintain Informal Games and Sports

In a study of childhood activity patterns, two social psychologists have noted that the television-viewing time of middle-class North American children has increased "in direct proportion to the efforts adults [have made] to involve them in organized activities" (Sherif & Rattray, 1976, p. 102). The inference underlying this observation is that adults may be wasting their time and money organizing sport programs for children because the programs interfere with learning how to actively organize informal games and sports. This case has been made by others as well. Devereaux (1976) has suggested that organized sport programs create a negative condition he calls "little leaguism." This condition, says Devereaux, robs children of valuable learning experiences because it undermines informal games. Historical surveys showing a decline in the number of informal games played by children in both the United States and England supports Devereaux's contention (Goodman, 1979; Opie & Opie, 1969). Other indirect support is found in studies showing that participation in informal games is less characteristic among middle- and upper income children than it is among children from lower socioeconomic backgrounds (Medrich et al., 1982). Organized sport programs are much more common in middle- and upper income neighborhoods than in low-income neighborhoods.

However, some research suggests that the existence of organized sport programs is not always associated with low rates of participation in informal games (Kleiber & Roberts, 1983; Medrich et al., 1982). In fact, in some cases the children who have participated the longest in organized sport programs have the highest rates of participation in informal games. One explanation for these findings is that many children may participate in informal games for the same reasons they participate in organized sport programs year after year. Another explanation is that participation in organized programs could actually provide young people with a knowledge of game models that could be used to initiate and sustain activities on their own.

In my own work on this topic I have observed that some children can use their experiences in organized programs as a starting point for getting together with friends and making up their own versions of games. But other children who have had the same experiences in organized programs do not seem to have the faintest idea about how to create games on their own. In the latter case, experiences in organized sports may have prevented young people from developing crucial organizational skills, or their experiences may have led them to define informal games as second-rate because such games are not "real." In other words, without uniforms, referees, coaches, nine players on each team, and a nicely lined field, these children have a difficult time playing what they have come to know as baseball.

In summary, the idea that organized sport programs undermine the informal games of children needs to be explored further. At this time, the data suggest that adults should be careful not to inadvertently discourage children from getting together and playing games on their own. Promoting involvement in organized programs should never be done at the expense of informal games and sports.

## Organized Sport Programs and Children's Play Values

Past research has led many sport scientists to conclude that participation in organized sport programs leads children to develop a "professional attitude" about their games (Kidd & Woodman, 1975; Mantel & Vander Velden, 1974; Webb, 1969). In other words, children learn to become more concerned with winning and playing well than with being fair and having fun. However, some good reasons exist for questioning this conclusion.

First, organized sport programs probably attract children who enjoy the challenge of goal-oriented activities. Therefore, these children are expected to score higher than others on any scale measuring so-called professional attitudes—not because of their experiences in the programs but because of the orientations they brought to the programs. Second, organized sport programs are intentionally designed to emphasize winning and playing well. Children realize this. When they become a part of those programs they quickly give high priority to these things. This does not necessarily mean they have abandoned their commitment to fairness or having fun. But in the organized programs they do not have to worry about fairness because the referees and the coaches take care of rules and rule enforcement. Furthermore, when they participate in the organized programs they may define fun in terms of playing well and winning. This does not mean that they have forever abandoned other definitions of fun; it only means that their definitions are somewhat flexible, and they can be changed to fit the demands of new situations.

The big question is whether taking fairness for granted and defining fun in terms of performance and winning carries over to informal games and interferes with the way these games are played. Carryover may occur for a few children (Podilchak, 1982), but no data indicates that the children who participate in organized sport programs become so obsessed with winning and playing well that it interferes with what goes on apart from organized sports. This also means that when children become overconcerned with winning and playing well in their organized sport programs, they need to change the programs themselves and the orientations of the adults who control them.

## Coaches' Influence on Children's Socialization Experiences in Organized Sport Programs

Although the coaches in organized youth sport programs have often been singled out for criticism, research shows that they are generally concerned with helping the players on their teams have fun and experience positive socialization outcomes (Weiss & Sisley, 1984). Research also shows that they do in fact have an impact on how children perceive and evaluate their personal experiences in the organized programs, the sports being played, and the teams for which they play (Harris, 1983, 1984; Smoll & Smith, 1980; Smoll, Smith, Curtis, & Hunt, 1978).

Not all coaches are perceived in exactly the same manner by their players. However, when they act in a punitive and critical manner they tend to be viewed negatively by the children on their teams. When they engage in supportive, teaching-oriented behaviors, they tend to be viewed positively. For many players, especially those lacking self-esteem or playing a sport for the first time, these evaluations of coaches are tied to how they evaluate their teams and the sport they are playing. This means that coaches must be able to provide supportive feedback in the form of guidance and instruction without criticizing their players in a negative manner and without using punishment as an instructional tool or as a means of social control.

This sounds like easy advice to follow, but research has shown that coaches often misperceive how their behavior affects the players on their teams (Martens & Simon, 1976; Smoll & Smith, 1980). When this happens children may experience socialization outcomes quite different than what coaches expect or intend. What may be needed to correct this situation are training programs designed to help coaches increase their awareness of how they affect the players on their youth sport teams. Research indicates that such programs can be effective (Smith, Smoll, & Curtis, 1979; Smith, Smoll, & Hunt, 1977).

Although we do know that coaches have an impact on how children define their sport experiences, we have no data on the extent to which coaches shape characteristics and behaviors that transcend sport-related situations and influence the rest of a child's life. Research on the social influence process suggests that coaches are most likely to produce positive socialization outcomes for players with whom they develop close, personal relationships. When the player-coach relationship is characterized by emotional ties and when few other influential adults exist in a young player's life, a coach may become a "significant other" for that person (Snyder, 1970). However, this does not occur very often.

## WHAT CHILDREN ARE LOOKING FOR
## IN THEIR SPORT EXPERIENCES

Whenever researchers turn to the topic of socialization and children's sports, they tend to focus attention on what adults think should be happening in children's lives. Although most adults would say they want to be responsive to the interests and needs of young people, their responsiveness does not often go beyond lip service when it comes to setting up organized sport programs. This means that those programs are often designed to fit adult conceptions of the sport experience and the socialization outcomes adults think should be associated with participation. But what do children want from their sport experiences?

One way to answer this question is to simply ask the children themselves, and another way is to watch children when they have opportunities to organize their own sport activities. When this has been done, the findings have not been very surprising (Coakley, 1983, 1986b). Children are primarily interested in four things:

- action
- personal involvement in the action
- close scores and challenges matching their skills
- opportunities to reaffirm relationships with friends

The importance of each of these factors can be illustrated through a brief description of what goes on in an informal game.

Whenever children create their own games a good deal of effort is devoted to setting up rules that foster action. Most of the activity during their games occurs around the scoring area, and scores are so frequent that it is often impossible to keep track of any personal performance statistics. When children are asked about what is most fun in their informal sport experiences they emphasize action-related events like "hitting," "catching," "shooting," "scoring," and so forth. Furthermore, sitting on the bench does not occur in informal games.

Rule qualifications and handicap systems are often developed to maximize the personal involvement of all participants and to sustain satisfying action. "Do-overs," "interference calls," and other special rules may be used to help less skilled players maintain their involvement at satisfying levels. The highly skilled players may assume leadership roles and develop creative strategies and personal responses that will help them maintain their own involvement at satisfying levels.

When organizing their own games children are quick to realize that close scores make games exciting and lopsided scores make them boring. Their games reflect this realization. Teams are often constructed or modified to keep game scores close enough to make the games interesting and challenging, even if individual players must accept handicaps like batting left-handed.

Finally, children use games to reaffirm their relationships with friends. The makeup of teams and the strategies they use during games reflect this desire. In fact, close scores may sometimes even be sacrificed in order to use games to reaffirm friendships.

When talking to children about their sport involvement and watching them play informal sports, it is clear that they are not interested in the socialization implications of their activities. In fact, character building is irrelevant in their games. However, one explanation for why action, involvement, close scores, and friendships are so important in children's informal sports is that children are basically interested in expressing themselves, learning new things about their own capabilities, and being recognized for demonstrating their skills. They set up their own sports so that these things happen very frequently.

The adults who work with youth sport programs would be wise to use what they know about children's informal sports to guide their attempts to organize those programs to meet the needs of young people. If children enjoy what happens in their organized sport experiences, they are more likely to be favorably influenced by the relationships occasioned by their participation. The task for adults is to keep the door open for the establishment of relationships through which socialization outcomes can occur. This is quite different from trying to organize programs so that lessons are somehow learned automatically through participation.

If the informal sports of children are used as a guide for making changes, recommendations for organized sport programs include the following:

• Make changes in games and game rules so that action is increased.

• Make changes in games and game rules so that the personal involvement of every player is increased.

• Make changes in game rules and scoring methods so that game scores are kept close and challenges are heightened.

• Change the ways teams are organized and the way practices are organized so that friends have opportunities to play together in a variety of ways.

Converting these recommendations into actual policies is amazingly easy if the game models used in youth sports programs are defined as arbitrary and changeable. Many adults have a difficult time doing this, but no divine messages have destined children's games to look forever like the games played by older athletes. Game models are not sacred. For example, the dimensions of playing areas can be altered, as can the size and weight of playing equipment. Rules can be changed, scoring can be promoted, scores can be kept close through rule changes and handicap systems, rosters can be designed to encourage the the reaffirmation of friendships, and practices can be organized to promote and nurture the development of friendships. Once game models are seen simply as tools for providing children with enjoyable experiences, the possibilities for change are endless (cf Coakley, 1986b; Hutslar, 1985).

Adults should remember that one of the things that makes sport participation so attractive in their own lives is that it has little meaning beyond the situations in which it occurs. Adults play games and matches having no implications for their family relationships, their occupational careers, financial status, or moral worth. Their involvement creates excitement and emotional arousal without involving any seriousness going beyond the activities themselves. This does not mean that sport involvement is not a potential source of learning for adults. In fact, what it does mean is that sport participation provides people with unique settings for their relationships with others, and those relationships can take on new dimensions that may not develop in other settings. This opens the doors for new experiences and new growth. It happens the same way for children. But because children are more impressionable than adults, such new experiences can happen more frequently and have more of an impact on their lives.

Adults should also remember that socialization outcomes are most likely to be positive when experiences are defined in favorable ways. Despite the old adage that people supposedly learn lessons from painful experiences, children are most likely to learn from experiences they enjoy and that lead to the development of close, expressive relationships with peers and with adult role models. Of course, the parents and coaches who are associated with youth sport programs must relate with program participants in meaningful ways, and they must communicate information to those participants through the example of their own behaviors.

## SUMMARY AND CONCLUSIONS

Children in most industrialized countries are introduced to organized sports early in their lives. However, their access to equipment, facilities, socialization experiences, and opportunities to participate vary with the socioeconomic status of their families, different types of family structures, race, and gender. Socialization into sports is strongly influenced by three factors: opportunities to participate, support from significant others, and a perception of self as a potential participant.

The consequences of sport participation are grounded in the social relationships occasioned by involvement. Socialization outcomes are most likely shaped by close, expressive relationships with fellow participants and with the adults who work in organized programs. Many people assume that participation in organized sport programs systematically produces positive socialization outcomes. They believe this because they are unaware of the selection processes associated with those programs, because they focus on the most outstanding young people who participate in the programs, and because sport provides them with unique opportunities to see young people display attributes that may have been developed through normal maturational processes apart from sport participation.

Parent-child relationships can be affected either positively or negatively as a result of the interaction associated with sport involvement. When parents use their children's sport involvement as a source of common interests, their relationships are likely to be enhanced. But when children perceive pressure from their parents, relationships are likely to be jeopardized.

Although the relationship between participation in organized sport programs and in informal games is not clear, children may come to overdepend on adults for guidance and supervision of their physical activities. In light of this adults should encourage participation in both types of settings. This conclusion is supported by information showing that the practices and games in organized programs are quite different from the games in informal sports (Coakley, 1983, 1986b). The former tend to be rule-centered and product-oriented whereas the latter tend to be action-centered and process-oriented. Because of this fact, the potential socialization outcomes of each are different, and both types of settings provide young people with valuable opportunities to learn things through their relationships with the other people involved.

Participation in organized sport programs probably does not lead children to value winning more than playing fair or having fun. However, organized programs are set up so that the children themselves do not have to be concerned with the development and enforcement of rules. Adults take care of those things. Children tend to develop definitions of fun that emphasize performance and game outcomes, at least while they are participating in organized sports. But no evidence suggests that these definitions carry over into other settings and preclude defining fun in other ways.

Coaches do have an impact on the players on their youth sport teams but probably not related to much more than how children perceive their sport experiences, the sports they are playing, and their teams. In some cases, coaches may become significant others in the lives of young people, but this outcome usually only occurs when they develop close, expressive relationships with children who lack role models and other adult sources of guidance and feedback. However, having an impact on the way young people define their sport experiences can have important long-term consequences for sport involvement patterns. This in itself makes coaches and coaching behaviors important components of the sport socialization process.

Finally, information on what children are looking for in their sport experiences suggests that they want action, personal involvement, close scores and challenges, and opportunities to reaffirm their friendships. Although no data exist on this issue, positive socialization outcomes seem to be maximized when the organized sport experiences of children provide them with these four things. Numerous changes could be made in existing organized programs to promote the things children want. Making these changes simply enhances the likelihood that children will develop the kind of relationships that will lead to a high socialization potential.

## REFERENCES

Ash, M.J. (1978). The role of research in children's competitive athletics. In R.A. Magill, M.J. Ash, & F.L. Smoll (Eds.), *Children in sport* (pp. 175–191). Champaign, IL: Human Kinetics.

Berlage, G. (1982). Children's sports and the family. *Arena Review,* **6**(1), 43–47.

Braddock, J. (1980, spring). Race, sports and social mobility: A critical review. *Sociological Symposium, 30*, 18–38.

Caplan, P.J. (1981). *Barriers between women*. Jamaica, NY: Spectrum Publications.

Chafetz, J.S. (1978). *Masculine, feminine, or human?* Itasca, IL: F.E. Peacock.

Coakley, J. (1983). Play, games, and sport: Developmental implications for young people. In J.C. Harris & R.J. Park (Eds.), *Play, games and sports in cultural contexts* (pp. 431–450). Champaign, IL: Human Kinetics.

Coakley, J. (1986a). Socialization and youth sports. In A. Miracle & C.R. Rees (Eds.), *Sport and social theory* (pp. 135–147). Champaign, IL: Human Kinetics.

Coakley, J. (1986b). *Sport in society: Issues and controversies* (3rd ed.). St. Louis, MO: C.V. Mosby.

Coakley, J., & Bredemeier, B. (1985, May). *Youth sports: Development of ethical practices*. Paper presented at the Ethics and Athletics Conference, Baton Rouge, LA.

Devereaux, E. (1976). Backyard versus Little League baseball: The impoverishment of children's games. In D. Landers (Ed.), *Social problems in athletics* (pp. 37–56). Urbana: University of Illinois Press.

Goodman, C. (1979). *Choosing sides*. New York: Shocken Books.

Harris, J.C. (1983). Interpreting youth baseball: Players' understandings of attention, winning, and playing the game. *Research Quarterly for Exercise and Sport, 54*(4), 330–339.

Harris, J.C. (1984). Interpreting youth baseball: Players' understandings of fun and excitement, danger and boredom. *Research Quarterly for Exercise and Sport, 55*(4), 379–382.

Harris, O., & Hunt, L. (1984). *Race and sports involvement: Some implications of sports for black and white youth*. Paper presented at the meetings of the American Alliance for Health, Physical Education, Recreation, and Dance, Anaheim, CA.

Hutslar, J. (1985). *Beyond Xs and Os*. Welcome, NC: Wooten.

Kidd, T.R., & Woodman, W. (1975). Sex and orientations toward winning in sport. *Research Quarterly, 46*(4), 476–483.

Kleiber, D., & Kelly, J. (1980). Leisure, socialization and the life cycle. In S. Iso-Ahola (Ed.), *Social psychological perspectives on leisure and recreation* (pp. 91–137). Springfield, IL: Charles C. Thomas.

Kleiber, D., & Roberts, G. (1983). The relationship between game and sport involvement in later childhood: A preliminary investigation. *Research Quarterly for Exercise and Sport, 54*(2), 200–203.

Lever, J. (1976). Sex differences in the games children play. *Social Problems,* **23**, 478–487.

Lever, J. (1978). Sex differences in the complexity of children's games. *American Sociological Review,* **43**(4), 471–483.

Lewis, M. (1972a). Culture and gender roles: There is no unisex in the nursery. *Psychology Today,* **5**(12), 54–57.

Lewis, M. (1972b). Sex differences in the play behavior of the very young. *Journal of Physical Education and Recreation,* **43**(6), 38–39.

Loy, J., McPherson, B.D., & Kenyon, G. (1978). *Sport and social systems.* Reading, MA: Addison-Wesley.

Mantel, R., & Vander Velden, L. (1974). The relationship between the professionalization of attitude toward play of preadolescent boys and participation in organized sport. In G.H. Sage (Ed.), *Sport and American society* (pp. 172–178). Reading, MA: Addison-Wesley.

Martens, R., & Simon, J. (1976). Comparison of three predictors of state anxiety in competitive situations. *Research Quarterly,* **47**, 381–387.

McGuire, R., & Cook, D. (1983). The influence of others and the decision to participate in youth sports. *Journal of Sport Behavior,* **6**(1), 9–16.

McPherson, B.D. (1985). Socialization theory and research: Toward a "new wave" of scholarly inquiry in a sport context. In A. Miracle & C.R. Rees (Eds.), *Sport and social theory* (pp. 111–134). Champaign, IL: Human Kinetics.

Medrich, E., Roizen, J., Rubin, V., Buckley, S. (1982). *The serious business of growing up.* Berkeley: University of California Press.

*Miller Lite report on American attitudes toward sports.* (1983). Milwaukee, WI: Miller Brewing Co. (Survey done by Research & Forecasts, Inc., New York)

Oliver, M. (1980). Race, class and the family's orientation to mobility through sport. *Sociological Symposium,* **30**, 62–86.

Opie, I., & Opie, P. (1969). *Children's games in street and playground.* Fair Lawn, NJ: Oxford University Press.

Orlick, T., & Botterill, C. (1975). *Every kid can win.* Chicago: Nelson-Hall.

Podilchak, W. (1982). Youth sport involvement: Impact on informal game participation. In A.O. Dunleavy, A.W. Miracle, & C.R. Rees (Eds.), *Studies in the sociology of sport* (pp. 325–348). Fort Worth: Texas Christian University Press.

Roberts, G., Kleiber, D., & Duda, J. (1981). An analysis of motivation in children's sport: The role of perceived competence in participation. *Journal of Sport Psychology,* **3**(3), 206–216.

Scanlon, T., & Lewthwaite, R. (1984). Social psychological aspects of competition for male youth sport participants: Vol. 1. Predictors of competitive stress. *Journal of Sport Psychology, 6*(2), 208–226.

Sherif, C., & Rattray, G. (1976). Psychological development and activity in middle childhood (5–12 years). In J. Albinson & G. Andrews (Eds.), *Child in sport and physical activity* (pp. 97–132). Baltimore, MD: University Park Press.

Smith, R.E., Smoll, F.L., & Curtis, B. (1979). Coach effectiveness training: A cognitive-behavioral approach to enhancing relationship skills in youth sport coaches. *Journal of Sport Psychology, 1*, 59–75.

Smith, R.E, Smoll, F.L., & Hunt, E.A. (1977). A system for the behavioral assessment of athletic coaches. *Research Quarterly, 48*, 401–407.

Smoll, F.L., & Smith, R.E. (1980). Techniques for improving self-awareness of youth sports coaches. *Journal of Physical Education and Recreation, 51*(2), 46–49, 52.

Smoll, F.L., Smith, R.E., Curtis, B., & Hunt, E. (1978). Toward a mediational model of coach-player relationships. *Research Quarterly, 49*, 528–541.

Snyder, E. (1970). Aspects of socialization in sports and physical education. *Quest, 14*, 1–7.

Snyder, E., & Purdy, D. (1982). Socialization into sport: Parent and child reverse and reciprocal effects. *Research Quarterly for Exercise and Sport, 53*(3), 263–266.

State of Michigan. (1978). *Joint Legislative study on youth sports programs*. A report presented to the Michigan State Legislature.

Watson, G. (1977). Games, socialization and parental values: Social class differences in parental evaluation of Little League baseball. *International Review of Sport Sociology, 12*(1), 17–47.

Webb, H. (1969). Professionalization of attitudes toward play among adolescents. In G. Kenyon (Ed.), *Aspects of contemporary sport sociology* (pp. 161–178). North Palm Beach, FL: The Athletic Institute.

Weiss, M., & Sisley, B. (1984). Where have all the coaches gone? *Sociology of Sport Journal, 1*(4), 332–347.

Yablonsky, L., & Brower, J. (1979). *The Little League game*. New York: Times Books.

# 4

# Understanding Attrition in Children's Sport

**Daniel Gould**

Children's sport involves a large and important segment of contemporary society. In the United States, for example, 17 million children between the ages of 6 and 16 are estimated to participate in more than 30 non-school-sponsored sport programs (Martens, 1986). From a worldwide perspective, if only 20% of the 640 million children in the world between the ages of 5 and 14 are involved in organized sport, this represents a phenomenal 128 million young lives.[1] Statistics alone make children's sport one of the most important childhood activities.

Paradoxically, although the large number of children participating in sport makes it a tremendous success, the attrition rate in these programs is an area of increasing concern. In an extensive study of sport participation patterns of children between the ages of 11 and 18, investigators from the State of Michigan's Youth Sport Institute found an attrition rate of 35% (Sapp & Haubenstricker, 1978). In a similar study of Australian schoolchildren, Robertson (1981) found an even higher attrition rate of 59%, whereas Pooley (1981) found an attrition rate of 22% in Canadian youth soccer players, and Sefton and Fry (1981) found a 35% rate for Canadian age-group swimmers. Lastly, Fry, McClements, and

Sefton (1981) have provided evidence that attrition rates in youth sports may be on the increase with the dropout rate for first-year youth ice hockey players increasing from 29 to 37% over a 6-year period.

Averaged together these descriptive findings reveal that approximately 35% of those involved in youth sport discontinue involvement each year. Even if many of these children return to participation after discontinuing initial involvement, millions of children still permanently drop out of sport. These staggering statistics have alarmed pediatric behavioral scientists, especially in light of the general conclusion that children's sport, when conducted properly, have beneficial effects on those who participate (Gould, in press; Martens, 1978; Martens & Seefeldt, 1979). For this reason, investigators have turned their attention to this important topic.

Pediatric sport scientists studying reasons for attrition in children's sport have arrived at different conclusions. Some (Feigley, 1984; Orlick, 1973; Orlick & Botterill, 1975; Pooley, 1981) have concluded that the high attrition rates result from an overemphasis on competition, burnout from overtraining, and inadequate organization and instruction. Others, such as Nettleton (1979), have suggested that few organizations can retain the interest of even 25 to 30% of their clientele over time and that the high attrition rates in youth sports are not unexpected. Still others (Gould & Horn, 1984; Guppy as cited in McPherson, Guppy, & McKay, 1976) have concluded that most children are not discontinuing sport involvement completely but are either discontinuing on a short-term basis or dropping out of one sport and entering another. Given the infancy of this line of research, a need exists to examine these issues.

The present review examines the children's sport attrition research and has a four-fold purpose. First, the descriptive studies assessing reasons for youth sport withdrawal will be reviewed to determine the current state of knowledge in the area. Second, the newly emerging studies designed to identify theoretically based motives for sport withdrawal will be examined. Third, a conceptual framework or model of youth sport withdrawal will be developed. This model will organize and integrate the previously discussed descriptive and theoretical research and show that by integrating these findings our understanding of attrition in children's sport is enhanced. Finally, based on an examination of the model, future research directions and practical implications will be outlined.

## DESCRIPTIVE STUDIES OF YOUTH SPORT WITHDRAWAL

Assessing children's motives for sport withdrawal is a relatively new area of research, with the first studies on the topic appearing in the early 1970s. Since the publication of these initial studies, however, more investigators have become interested in the area, and a body of literature has begun to evolve. More importantly, consistent patterns of findings have begun to emerge across studies.

The first investigation of the youth sport dropout was conducted by Orlick (1973). In this study, 32 Canadian children, aged 8 to 9 and who had withdrawn from organized sports, participated in open-ended interviews. Orlick concluded that lack of participation, fear of failure, disapproval by significant others, and psychological stress were the underlying factors for the children's decisions to withdraw from competitive sport. He also suggested that when children of this age discontinue sport participation, they are reacting to a negative environment created from the emphasis of coaches and the structure of the sports themselves.

Orlick and Botterill conducted a second investigation (Orlick, 1974; Orlick & Botterill, 1975), designed to examine further reasons for children's sport withdrawal. They extensively interviewed 60 former sport participants ranging in age from 7 to 19 years and representing baseball, cross-country skiing, ice hockey, soccer, and swimming. The findings revealed that 40 of the 60 subjects (67%) withdrew because of program emphasis. Thirty of these 40 children discontinued because of the competitive nature of the program, citing their lack of enjoyment, the seriousness of the sport, and the emphasis on winning as major motives for withdrawal. The remaining 10 children indicated that they had discontinued because of coaches' actions, which included such things as leaving players out of contests, criticizing players frequently, and pushing the athletes too hard. Twenty-one percent of the 60 former participants indicated that they discontinued participation because of conflicts of interest with nonsport activities, 10% because of interest in other sports, and 2% because of injury. Finally, reasons for discontinuing were found to be age-related as 60% of the high school–aged dropouts withdrew because of conflicting sport and nonsport interests, whereas all the elementary school–aged dropouts discontinued either because of little success (60%) or a lack of playing time.

The studies by Orlick and Orlick and Botterill provided valuable initial information about children's motives for sport withdrawal. These initial efforts, however, were characterized by small samples and focused exclusively on qualitative data analyses. In contrast, Sapp and Haubenstricker's (1978) and Robertson's (1981) investigations of the youth sport dropout were much larger in scope, whereas Petlichkoff (1982) used both descriptive and inferential statistics in her investigation of the youth sport dropout.

In the Sapp and Haubenstricker (1978) investigation, 1,183 male and female active athletes aged 11 to 18 years and parents of 418 athletes aged 6 to 10 years completed a survey assessing both participation motives and reasons for sport withdrawal. These young athletes and parents represented a wide variety of sports including baseball, softball, basketball, bowling, tackle football, golf, figure skating, gymnastics, ice hockey, soccer, swimming, synchronized swimming, tennis, track and field, and wrestling. Thirty-five percent of the older athletes and 24% of the parents of the younger athletes indicated that they or their children did not plan to participate in the next season. Of the athletes who indicated that they did not plan to participate next season, 64% rated involvement in other activities, 44% rated working, and 34% rated disinterest as the major motives for dropping out. Less than 15% of the athletes rated lack of participation, dislike of the coach, injury, expense, and dislike for teammates as important. Sixty-five percent of the parents of younger athletes who indicated that their children would no longer participate also reported involvement in other activities as the most frequent reason for their children discontinuing involvement, whereas 43% indicated that their children were not interested in the sport.[2]

Robertson's (1981) study involved the assessment of reasons for discontinuing sport participation in 405 male and 353 female 12-year-old, Australian former athletes. The results revealed that 51% of the boys and 39% of the girls discontinued because of the program emphasis (e.g., "boring," "no fun," "never played", "too rough", "not interested"); 14% of the boys and 17% of the girls rated general life conflicts (e.g., "no free time", "social life", "got a job"); and 12% of the boys and 1% of the girls rated other sport conflicts as major motives for withdrawal.

In her study, Petlichkoff (1982) surveyed 46 former junior high and high school athletes aged 12 to 18 and found that having other things to do (78%); being injured (58%); not improving skills (52%); not being as good as wanted to be (52%); and not having enough fun (52%) were the motives rated as being most important for discontinuing involvement. Younger dropouts were found to differ significantly from older dropouts, in that they rated different factors as more important for discontinuing. These included no teamwork, did not meet new friends, did not feel important enough, not challenged enough, and skills did not improve. Thus, the younger dropouts were suggested to be more socially oriented and hopeful their participation would lead to meeting new friends and gaining recognition. Follow-up interviews also revealed that 59% of the dropouts had not participated in any organized sport since discontinuing involvement.

The investigations reviewed thus far have focused on the assessment of motives for sport withdrawal in young athletes representing a variety of sports. Other investigators, however, have focused on assessing motives for sport withdrawal in former athletes from specific sports. In particular, Pooley (1981) examined dropouts in soccer; Fry, McClements, and Sefton (1981) in ice hockey; Gould, Feltz, Horn, and Weiss (1982) and Sefton and Fry (1981) in swimming; Robinson and Carron (1982) in football; Burton and Martens (1986) in wrestling; and Klint and Weiss (1986) in gymnastics.

Pooley (1981) conducted extensive interviews with 50 youth soccer dropouts, 10 to 15 years old. His results revealed that 54% of the children reported that they stopped playing because of conflicts of interest; 33% cited the overemphasis on competition (e.g., the coach shouted when errors were made); and 10% cited poor communication. Younger (10- to 12-year-old) as compared to older (13- to 15-year-old) participants were also found to withdraw more often because of the overemphasis on competition.

In an extensive study of youth hockey participants and dropouts, Fry, McClements, and Sefton (1981) surveyed 200 dropouts, aged 8 to 16. When asked why they stopped playing hockey these children indicated conflicts of interest (31%); lack of skill (15%); dislike of coach (14%); rough play (10%); and organizational difficulties (10%; e.g., inconvenient game times) as major motives for their decision to withdraw. Young players (under age 9) were also found to rate a lack of skill and no fun or boredom as more important motives for discontinuing than the older players. Dropouts were also found to demonstrate a lower achievement orientation than the active participants.

Gould et al. (1982) examined motives for attrition in 50 former swimmers 10 to 18 years old. Important motives for discontinuing were "other things to do" (rated as important by 49% of the respondents), "not enough fun" (28%), "wanted to participate in another sport" (24%), "not as good as wanted to be" (24%), "dislike of the coach" (20%), "did not like the pressure" (16%), "boredom" (16%), and "training too hard" (16%). Based on these findings, the researchers concluded that these former swimmers most often discontinued because of conflicts of interest (84% of the respondents rated this as an important or very important motive). However, a lack of ability, dislike of the coach, dislike of the pressure, boredom, and training too hard were, at times, important factors affecting the young swimmers' decision to withdraw from the sport.

Sefton and Fry (1981) also examined children's motives for discontinuing swimming in a cross-sectional study of active ($n = 72$) and former swimmers ($n = 86$), ranging in age from 6 to 22 years. The findings revealed that major motives for withdrawal included too much time (rated as important by 31% of the former swimmers); dissatisfaction with practices (27%); conflicts with other activities (14%); favoritism displayed by coaches (12%); an overdemanding coach (12%); injuries (9%); and work (9%). Sixty-seven percent of the former swimmers also reported that they achieved what they had hoped from competitive swimming, whereas 30% said they did not. Fifty-eight percent of the former swimmers indicated that they would never swim competitively again, whereas 42% thought they would. Finally, when asked what changes they would make in competitive swimming before participating again, 19% of the former swimmers cited reduced practice time; 8% a more understanding coach; and 6% more variety in practices.

One of the best designed studies examining youth sport dropouts was conducted by Robinson and Carron (1982). These investigators adopted a Lewinian interactionist framework where dropout behavior was viewed as a product of both personal and environmental factors (Lewin, 1935). A variety of personal and situational factors was then selected as variables thought to influence sport withdrawal. These included competitive trait anxiety, achievement motivation, self-motivation, self-esteem, causal attributions, attitudes toward competition, sportsmanship, communication measures, parental and group sport involvement, coach leadership, and group cohesion. These variables were assessed in 98 high school football players who were classified as either football dropouts ($n = 26$), football starters ($n$ = 33), or football survivors or nonstarters ($n$ = 39). The results supported the interactionist model as both situational and personal factors discriminated between the groups. In particular, dropouts were found to feel less a part of the team, enjoyed participation less, felt they had less support from their fathers for participation, more often attributed poor performance to ability, less often attributed success to effort, and more often viewed the coach as an autocrat than the other groups, who also differed from one another.

Robinson and Carron's (1982) investigation is important as it further supports the notion that the youth sport attrition process is a complex phenomenon influenced by a variety of personal and situational variables. Based on these findings and those of the previously reviewed studies, an interactionist framework must be adopted if attrition in children's sport is to be fully understood.

Youth wrestlers and former wrestlers aged 7 to 17 were the focus of a recent investigation by Burton and Martens (1986). Eighty-three youth wrestlers, 83 parents of these wrestlers, 26 former wrestlers, 26 parents of the former wrestlers, and 69 coaches were asked to rate reasons why children discontinue wrestling. The results revealed that "other things to do" was the major motive cited for discontinuing by all five groups. Other motives rated as important included "doesn't care any more," "no fun," and "isn't motivated any more." Although certain patterns of attrition motives were evident over all groups, considerable variation occurred between the groups in their ratings of motives for sport withdrawal.

Finally, Klint and Weiss (1986) examined participant motives in 43 competitive gymnasts, 26 recreational gymnasts, and 37 former competitive gymnasts. Each of these groups were surveyed regarding their reasons for participating in gymnastics, and the former gymnasts were also interviewed regarding why they discontinued gymnastics involvement. When motives for participation were examined, the competitive gymnasts most often cited fitness and challenge; the recreational gymnasts cited fun and situational factors (e.g., like to use the equipment); and the former gymnasts cited fun, challenge, and action as the most important motives for involvement. The former gymnasts also indicated that they most often discontinued involvement because they had other things to do, did not like the pressure, did not have enough fun, and felt gymnastics required too much time. When asked to indicate the single most important reason for withdrawing from gymnastics, 19% of the former gymnasts cited injury; 14% not enough fun, 11% dislike of the pressure, and 11% too much time. Only 2 of the 37 former gymnasts studied discontinued sport participation completely. After initially dropping out, the remaining 35 individuals either returned to gymnastics at a different level or became involved in other sports.

A number of general conclusions can be derived from these descriptive studies examining motives for youth sport withdrawal. Former youth sport participants cite a number of varied personal and situational reasons for sport withdrawal. These include such diverse motives as interest in other activities, conflicts of interest, lack of playing time, lack of success, little skill improvement, lack of fun, boredom, and injury. Conflicts of interest and interest in other activities have been found to be the most consistently cited motives for sport withdrawal. Other more negative motives such as a lack of playing time, overemphasis on competition, boredom, competitive stress, dislike of the coach, and no fun have been rated as major motives for sport withdrawal by a smaller number of former participants. Some evidence reveals that these more negative motives play a more important role in the discontinuation of younger as compared to older dropouts. Several studies have shown that most young athletes who discontinue participation do not totally withdraw from sport. In contrast, they reenter the same sport or participate in other sports at some time in the future.

## THEORETICAL ATTEMPTS TO EXAMINE YOUTH SPORT WITHDRAWAL

This review has shown that the majority of the youth sport attrition studies conducted to date have been descriptive in nature. These studies helped to identify important trends and variables influencing the attrition process. However, descriptive studies alone will not further advance knowledge in the area. Theoretical or conceptual models are needed that allow researchers to explain and predict behavior. For example, the descriptive research has clearly shown that large numbers of children discontinue involvement because of interest in or conflicts of interest with other activities. What has not been shown in these studies, however, is whether the changing of children's interests from one sport to another or from sport to nonsport activities results from a normal trial-and-error sampling process that allows children to identify activities that they most like, or whether it reflects the inability of organized sport programs to meet the psychological needs of a high percentage of children (Burton & Martens, 1985). This question has prompted investigators to begin to search for various theoretical constructs that may underlie a child's decision to discontinue sport involvement.

Thus, the time has come to go beyond descriptive studies of attrition in youth sports and to begin to develop theoretical models to explain the attrition process. To date, three theoretical frameworks have been identified as possible explanations of the underlying causes of attrition in children's sport. These include the achievement orientation, competence motivation, and social exchange/cognitive-affective frameworks.

### Achievement Orientation Theory

Ewing (1981) and Roberts (1984) were two of the first investigators to examine attrition in children's sport from a conceptual framework. These investigators used Maehr and Nicholls's (1980) cognitive interpretation of achievement motivation theory to explain youth sport persistence and withdrawal. They contended that in order to fully understand achievement behavior, the child's perception of success and failure, as well as his or her achievement goals, must also be understood. In essence, three orientations or goals of achievement behavior are said to exist: (a) an ability orientation where a child participates in an activity in an effort to demonstrate high ability and minimize low ability, usually by winning; (b) a task orientation where the child participates in an effort to perform the task as well as possible, regardless of any competitive outcome; and (c) a social approval orientation where the child participates in an effort to seek approval from significant others, usually by exhibiting maximum effort. These multiple goals of achievement are important because the extent to which a child will be motivated and remain active in an achievement context (e.g., sport) depends on his or her perception of whether his or her achievement goals are satisfied. Thus, to predict sport persistence and withdrawal, researchers must determine the salient achievement orientations of the child and the degree to which the child perceives that these achievement goals are fulfilled.

Based on this achievement orientation framework, Ewing (1981) predicted that individual differences in achievement orientations will emerge in children and that these differences in orientation will be related to both youth sport participation and withdrawal. Specifically, ability, task, and social approval orientations were predicted to emerge when young athletes were asked to identify their motives for participation. Children who were more ability oriented were expected to persist longer in sport (be athletes) than children who were not as high on ability orientation (nonparticipants or dropouts). In order to test these predicted achievement goals, perceived sport success, perceived sport failure, and attributions were assessed in 452 males and females who were 14 to 15 years old and who had been identified as sport participants, nonparticipants, or dropouts. The results supported the theory's prediction that multiple achievement goals would exist, in that ability and social approval orientations clearly emerged on a factor analysis, although no clear task orientation was identified. In addition, a relationship was found between achievement orientations, sport persistence, and sport withdrawal. Contrary to the predictions, however, the active sport participants did not display a higher ability orientation than the dropouts or the nonparticipants. Instead, the active sport participants were characterized by a social approval orientation and dropouts by an ability orientation. It was suggested that social approval–oriented children persist longer in sport because the organized sport structure provides ample opportunities for social support (e.g., coaches, parents, and teammates reward their expenditure of maximum effort). For the ability-oriented dropouts, however, the organized sport structure exposed their performance limits (they demonstrated "low" ability by failing) or did not allow them ample opportunity to test their abilities (they sat on the bench). Consequently, the ability-oriented children's goal of demonstrating high ability by winning was not fulfilled, so they were more likely to discontinue participation.

Although Ewing's (1981) study provides some initial support for Maehr and Nicholls's (1980) theoretical contentions, to date it has been the only empirical study conducted on the topic, and its utility therefore cannot yet be judged. It has much intuitive appeal, however, in that it specifies that individual differences exist in achievement orientations of young athletes and that sport persistence is dependent on the fulfillment of these objectives. Additionally, this theoretical framework is parsimonious because it contends that children can be characterized by three general achievement orientations.

## Competence Motivation Theory

A second theoretical approach that has been used to explain attrition in youth sport is Harter's (1978) theory of competence motivation. Based on White's (1959) earlier theory, Harter (1978, 1981) predicted that children are motivated to experience mastery or competence feelings when dealing with their environment and because of this, they seek to demonstrate or acquire competencies by engaging in mastery attempts. When mastery is attained (e.g., they are successful), perceived competence is enhanced, which in turn increases competence motivation. Increased competence motivation then causes the child to seek out other situations where competence can be developed. Thus, young athletes who perceive themselves to be highly competent or confident at a particular skill will persist longer at the skill and maintain interest in mastering the skill. In contrast, individuals who perceive themselves to have low competence at a particular skill will not maintain task persistence and interest. Harter does not view perceived competence as being a global trait or unitary construct but rather as having specific domains in the areas of physical, social, and cognitive concerns. Quite possibly, then, a child could show variations in motivation across these competence domains depending on his or her history of experiences and socialization.

Not only does Harter's (1978) model explain the perceived competence and task persistence/performance relationship, but it also accounts for the development of competence. A history of success in mastering skills leads to perceived competence, which in turn leads to increased motivation to be competent. On the other hand, children who have had a history of unsuccessful mastery attempts in a given activity usually experience feelings of low competence. This perception of low competence in turn decreases their motivation to continue participation in that activity. Harter's model also suggests that children who have little experience in a given type of activity will not have had the opportunity to develop a sense of competence in that domain.

Harter's theory is not only intuitively appealing, but it seems directly applicable for researchers studying participation motivation in young athletes. Unfortunately, research has only begun to test its contentions in the athletic domain, although preliminary support for its predictions have been generated in academic classroom situations (Harter, 1978). Evidence also indirectly supports Harter's hypothesis that one's participation motivation is related to a history of successful mastery attempts, in that former young athletes indicated that a lack of success and a lack of skill improvement were important reasons for discontinuing their participation in competitive sports. No direct link can be made between these variables, however, because these studies have not directly assessed perceived competence as the possible mediating variable.

One of the few studies designed to directly test Harter's (1978) model in the area of sports was conducted by Roberts, Kleiber, and Duda (1981). Roberts and his colleagues used Harter's (1979) Perceived Competence Scale for Children to compare male and female fourth and fifth graders who were either participants or nonparticipants in organized sport. They hypothesized that children who participate in organized sport programs would be higher in perceived physical competence than nonparticipants. Their results revealed that the youth sport participants were not only higher in perceived physical competence, but in social competence and general self-worth as well. These findings suggested that either the experience of sport participation influences perceptions of competence or that children with high perceptions of competence are attracted to and persist in sport. To address this issue, Roberts and his associates examined the relationship between years of experience in sport and perceived competence. The nonsignificant correlations between perceived competence and years of experience suggested that individuals with higher perceptions of competence select sport as an activity to demonstrate their abilities. In using only fourth- and fifth-grade students, however, the limited range of years of experience in these subjects may have masked the possible influence that sport experience may have on the development of perceived competence.

A second study designed to examine perceived competence in a youth sport setting was conducted by Feltz, Gould, Horn, and Weiss (1982). This study examined the effects that gender and years of competitive swimming experience had on the perceived competence of young swimmers ($n = 349$) and former swimmers ($n = 50$). Differences between swimmers and former swimmers in perceived competence were also studied. Unlike the results of Roberts and his colleagues, significant (but low) correlations were found between length of swimming involvement and perceived physical and social competence. In addition, male dropouts were found to exhibit higher levels of perceived physical competence and general self-esteem than female dropouts. A limitation of the statistical analyses employed prohibited the desired comparison of participants and former participants.

Feltz and Petlichkoff (1983) examined the relationship among perceived physical competence, participation status (active athlete or dropout), years of athletic experience, and gender. The sample studied included 239 participants and 43 dropouts representing a number of school-sponsored sports. A significant but low relationship existed between perceived physical competence and length of sport participation. Moreover, active participants were found to exhibit significantly higher levels of perceived competence than dropouts and males higher levels of competence than females.

Finally, in a study related to competence motivation, Burton and Martens (1986) examined the relationship between young athletes' perception of their ability and the decision to drop out of sport. Unlike previous theorists who focused solely on the competence-persistence relationship, however, these investigators hypothesized that this relationship can only be understood if other factors are examined, such as the child's perception of success and failure, activity importance, and expectations of parents and coaches. A preliminary test of their hypotheses was conducted using the previously discussed sample of active youth wrestlers, parents of active wrestlers, wrestling dropouts, parents of wrestling dropouts, and coaches. Their results supported the notion that dropouts turn to other activities when wrestling no longer allows them opportunities to perceive themselves high in ability. Specifically, participants reported higher levels of perceived ability, were characterized by more positive future performance expectancies, and exhibited more realistic minimal acceptable standards of performance than the dropouts. Perceived ability, then, when examined in conjunction with these external factors, proved to be a strong predictor of persistence.

The studies examining the relationship between perceived competence (or ability) and sport persistence are encouraging. Dropouts have been consistently found to demonstrate lower levels of perceived competence than participants, and perceived competence seems to be related to years of experience. Additional studies are needed, however, to determine definitely whether children characterized by high levels of competence are drawn to sport in efforts to demonstrate mastery or whether sport participation fosters competence. Moreover, Weiss, Bredemeier, and Shewchuk (1986) have indicated that the competence-persistence relationship is mediated by three interrelated variables. These include the child's intrinsic-extrinsic motivational orientation, perceived control (the child's perception of who or what is responsible for success-failure), and actual achievement. The athletic dropout can only be better understood when the complex interaction among these variables is studied.

## Social Exchange and Cognitive-Affective Theories

Smith (1986) has proposed the most recent theoretical framework to explain the process of sport withdrawal. In this framework the important distinction is made between sport burnout and sport dropout. Specifically, burnout-induced withdrawal is defined as the psychological, emotional, and physical withdrawal from sport resulting from chronic stress, whereas dropping out results from a change of interests and/or value reorientation. Thus, all sport dropouts are not necessarily burnouts.

The distinction between the dropout and burnout is central to the conceptual framework forwarded by Smith (1986), who convincingly argues that the dropout and burnout syndromes have differing theoretical explanations. That is, a social exchange model best explains dropout forms of withdrawal, whereas a cognitive-affective model best explains athletic burnout.

Smith (1986) uses the classic social exchange framework developed by Thibaut and Kelly (1959) to explain the process of dropping out of sport. According to this theory, the decision to participate and persist in sport is a function of costs (e.g., time and effort, anxiety, disapproval of others) and benefits (e.g., trophies, feelings of competence) with the athlete constantly trying to maximize benefits and minimize costs. Thus, interest and participation is maintained when the benefits outweigh the costs, and withdrawal occurs when costs outweigh benefits. However, behavior is not fully explained by a simple rewards-minus-costs formula. The decision to participate and persist is mediated by the athlete's minimum comparison level (the lowest criteria one used to judge something as satisfying or unsatisfying) and the comparison level of alternative activities. Consequently, someone may choose to stay involved in sport even if costs are exceeded by rewards because no alternative opportunities are available. Similarly, an athlete who perceives that the rewards outweigh costs in a program may discontinue involvement because a more desirable alternative activity is available.

Although a direct empirical test for the social exchange interpretation of youth sport withdrawal has not been conducted, this formulation seems to readily explain the existing findings in the area (Smith, 1986). Participation motivation studies show that children are attracted to sport because of a variety of benefits and awards. Dropping out of sport occurs when children perceive costs to outweigh benefits and have other, desirable activities available. Hence, the most prevalent motive cited for discontinuing involvement is interest in other activities or conflicts of interest.

In contrast to the vast majority of individuals who drop out of sport, Smith (1986) argues that burnout does occur in a substantial minority of these athletes (and coaches). Athletes who burn out are often very successful, but the previously pleasurable activity becomes a source of undue stress as performance demands are perceived to outweigh one's capabilities. A lack of energy, exhaustion, sleeplessness, depression, tension, irritability, and anger often result. The situation becomes unbearable, and the athlete discontinues involvement as a method of coping with stress.

Smith (1986) has proposed a cognitive-affective model to explain the burnout process. This theoretical framework parallels his general model of athletic stress (Smith, 1986) and draws heavily upon the burnout literature from the social service professions. Figure 1 contains these models and shows that burnout occurs when the athlete perceives an imbalance between environmental

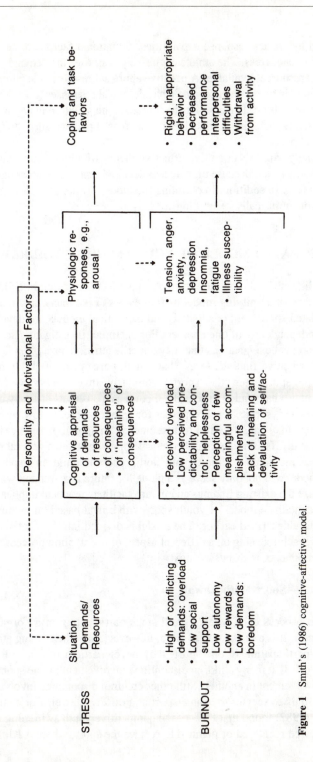

**Figure 1** Smith's (1986) cognitive-affective model.

demand and his or her response capabilities. Situational factors alone, however, do not create stress. The athlete cognitively appraises the demands of the situation and resources available. A negative appraisal results in the perception of threat, which in turn influences one's physiological responses (e.g., tension, fatigue). Finally, the athlete attempts to cope with the situation in any number of ways, possibly including rigid behavior, decreased performance, and withdrawal from sport.

Unfortunately, Smith's cognitive-affective theory of athletic stress has not been empirically tested because of its recent development. It has great intuitive appeal, however. In addition, in outlining the model, Smith provides specific guidelines for empirically examining it.

## AN INTEGRATED MODEL OF YOUTH SPORT WITHDRAWAL

One of the difficulties facing those trying to understand attrition in children's sport is the lack of a unifying model or framework. Like many new research areas, unrelated studies are conducted, and theoretical models are developed and tested independently of one another. For example, investigators studying possible theoretical explanations that may underlie attrition have often ignored important descriptive findings (e.g., that a high percentage of children who withdraw from sport enter other sports). Similarly, investigators conducting descriptive studies have failed to consider theoretical constructs that may underlie frequently cited, surface-level responses for withdrawal (e.g., low perceived ability feelings may cause a child to lose interest in sport). A need exists to integrate these diverse findings and theoretical approaches into a general model that describes and helps explain the attrition process in children's sport. An integrated model will not only serve as a guide for future research but will also better organize the existing findings and in turn facilitate practical implications.

Figure 2 contains a model of youth sport withdrawal based on an analysis of the literature described earlier. The model is divided into four interrelated components, each focusing on a different aspect of the attrition process. Each of these components is discussed next.

### Component 1—Sport Withdrawal

The attrition process ends when a child stops participating in an organized sports program. It is a mistake to assume, however, that when young athletes discontinue participation in one sport, they never participate again. Recent research reveals that many children discontinue involvement in one sport only to initiate involvement in another. Still other children discontinue involvement in one sport only to reenter the same sport at a different level. For example, Gould et al. (1982) found that 80% of the competitive youth swimming dropouts interviewed reentered or planned to reenter the sport, whereas Klint and

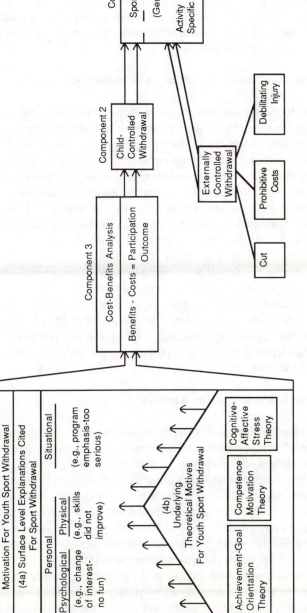

**Figure 2** A model of youth sport withdrawal.

Weiss (1986) found that 35 of 37 of the dropouts they surveyed reentered gymnastics or other sports. This is not to say that some children who drop out of sport never participate again. Petlichkoff (1982) found that 59% of the high school dropouts she interviewed had not participated in any organized sport since discontinuing involvement. Consequently, in Component 1 of the model, sport withdrawal is viewed on a continuum ranging from an activity-specific or program-specific withdrawal (e.g., drop out of baseball or a specific baseball program) to a domain-general withdrawal (e.g., drop out of all competitive sports permanently).

## Component 2—Child- or Externally Controlled Withdrawal

Working back from the actual decision to withdraw, the second component of the model focuses on whether young athletes control the decision to withdraw. In some cases, the decision to withdraw is externally controlled. For example, children who are cut from teams, can no longer afford the costs of some sports, or suffer such severe injuries that they are no longer able to participate have little choice about the decision to withdraw. Unfortunately, few studies have focused on this aspect of the attrition process, although Ogilvie and Howe (1982) have speculated that the ramifications of such withdrawal can be devastating. Especially significant would be studies examining the effects of "cutting" on the perceived competence and intrinsic motivation of the child.

Child-controlled withdrawal occurs more frequently than externally controlled withdrawal and has been the focus of most of the research conducted to date. In the case of child-controlled withdrawal, the young athlete makes the ultimate decision to discontinue participation. Even though the child makes the ultimate decision to discontinue, however, this decision can be markedly influenced by outside sources like the actions of coaches and parents and success or failure received in the program.

## Component 3—Costs-Benefits Analysis

The costs-benefits analysis that the child uses in making the decision to discontinue involvement is contained in Component 3. Based on Smith's (1986) application of the social exchange framework, the young athlete weighs the perceived benefits of participation against the costs, relative to his or her minimal comparison level (the minimum criteria he or she uses to define success or benefits) and the attractiveness and availability of alternative sport and nonsport activities (the comparison level for alternatives). In essence, when the child athlete perceives costs to outweigh benefits and alternative activities to be more attractive, he or she discontinues participation.

Smith's (1986) costs-benefits application of social exchange theory was separately incorporated in this component of the model because it provides a general theoretical framework that integrates both surface-level explanations cited for sport withdrawal, as well as underlying theoretical motives (see Component 4). Specifically, this framework predicts that children withdraw from sport when costs outweigh benefits, whether costs-benefits be defined as a young athlete's perceived competence, satisfaction of ability, task and social approval goals, psychological stress, or other varied personal and situational factors.

## Component 4—Motivation for Sport Withdrawal

Component 4 of the model is subdivided into two highly interrelated subcomponents. Subcomponent 4a depicts the surface-level explanations or self-ratings of program costs that children cite for discontinuing involvement. An interactionist paradigm is employed in this component, as the attrition research has shown that both personal and situational factors are cited as variables influencing the decision to withdraw. Personal reasons include psychological factors like interest in other activities, no fun, and competitive stress. Physical factors include such items as a lack of skill improvement and injury, and situational factors include things like program emphasis, poor organization, and social support from significant others. Finally, although the reasons cited for withdrawal are subdivided into categories, they do overlap considerably.

Subcomponent 4b of the model contains theoretical motives that underlie and affect the stated reasons for sport withdrawal. For example, a child may be unable to express whether she or he is task-, socially, or ability-oriented, yet individual differences exist on these achievement orientations and have been linked to participation persistence (Ewing, 1981). Similarly, the child's competence motivation or perceived competence has been shown to be an important variable affecting the attrition process, with dropouts being characterized by lower levels of competence than active participants. Finally, Smith's (1986) cognitive-affective model of athletic burnout seems especially appropriate for explaining attrition in a specific subclass of youth sport dropouts—those burnouts who suffer from the effects of chronic stress.

In summary, this model has the advantage of integrating both the descriptive and theoretical findings on attrition in children's sport. It is also broad in scope, integrating the social exchange, achievement orientation, perceived competence, and cognitive-affective theoretical frameworks. Finally, it emphasizes precisely defining the generality of youth sport withdrawal and the important distinction between dropouts and burnouts.

## FUTURE DIRECTIONS IN YOUTH SPORT ATTRITION RESEARCH AND PRACTICE

This review has clearly shown that much has been learned from the youth sport attrition research conducted to date. If further improvements are to be made, however, a number of theoretical, methodological, and measurement concerns must be addressed. Moreover, the conceptual model outlined in this review can serve as a guide for examining these research issues, as well as a guide for implementing practices designed to curtail attrition.

**Future Research Directions**

The youth sport attrition model outlined in Figure 2 clearly shows that to understand youth sport withdrawal, investigators must integrate the descriptive responses children give for dropping out of sport with possible underlying motivational constructs. In particular, Component 4 of the model shows that the achievement orientation, competence motivation, and cognitive-affective burnout theories all contain likely motives that may underlie sport withdrawal. Merely testing each theory's predictions with samples of active and former participants is not enough, however. Critical studies are needed in which these theories are tested simultaneously.

The need for designing critical investigations is especially noteworthy because the theories contained in the model are similar in many ways. For example, they are all cognitively oriented and focus on the child's perceptions of specified psychological or environmental states (e.g., perceived competence). Quite possibly, then, these theories are not comprised of independent psychological constructs and may at times discuss the same constructs under the guise of different labels. Thus, simultaneous tests of the various theories will determine if explanatory and predictive overlap exists.

Not only must varying theoretical constructs be simultaneously examined, but the model suggests that investigators should assess both theoretical and descriptive explanations for sport withdrawal. Investigators too often assume that the specific theoretical construct in which they are interested accounts for 100% of the variance in young athletes' decisions to withdraw. The research clearly shows, however, that the attrition process is complex and influenced by several factors. What is needed are studies that show how important various theoretically and practically grounded measures are in predicting withdrawal and when, in what situations, and with whom these measures explain and predict behavior.

Investigators utilizing this model will not only need to identify the underlying explanations for attrition in children's sport, but they must also stress the most advanced elements of theory—behavioral prediction and control. Yet, this review has shown that the majority of studies conducted to date have utilized a traditional field study paradigm where variables are observed but causal relationships not pursued. Consequently, causal inferences cannot be made. A need exists to conduct field experiments in which investigators test causal links between variables and behavior or to design studies that use path and structural-analytic statistical techniques that can be used to test causal links in nonexperimental settings. For example, Smith, Smoll, Hunt, Curtis, and Coppel (1979) have conducted a systematic series of studies that focus on how coaching behaviors influence the affective states of young athletes. A logical extension of this line of research would involve the assessment of young athletes' participation motives or achievement orientations. Coaching behaviors hypothesized to influence the various motives could also be assessed. The predicted correspondence between participation motives, coaching behaviors, attrition rates, and attrition motives could then be examined.

Components 1 and 2 of the model focus on identifying the extent and type of withdrawal that occur in youth sport. Future investigators must consider these components further because the lack of appropriate operational definitions has plagued the previous research. For example, little consistency has occurred across studies in regard to the definition of an athlete or dropout. Many of the previous studies have simply defined a dropout as a child who no longer participates in a particular sport. Component 1 of the model, however, reflects the finding that many of these children reenter sport. A dropout who reenters sport (an activity-specific dropout) may be considerably different from one who never returns (a domain-general dropout). Smith (1986) has also shown that an athletic burnout is substantially different from a dropout. Consequently, future investigators must heed the advice of investigators like Robinson and Carron (1982) and Smith (1986) and better define the participation-persistence continuum, including such levels as active athlete (starter), survivor (active athlete who receives little playing time), dropout, and burnout.

The model also reveals that two types of withdrawal can exist (see Component 2). Unfortunately, most of the existing research has focused solely on examining child-controlled withdrawal. Examining externally controlled withdrawal and its effects on future sport involvement is an important area for additional study.

The previous research has also been characterized by small, nonrandom samples. A need exists to ensure that minimal sample sizes and, when appropriate, random samples are obtained. Similarly, if many moderator variables are to be examined (e.g., gender, sport played, age, years of experience), samples should be selected that provide an adequate range of these variables.

Lastly, when conducting future investigations designed to assess costs and benefits of participation, as well as motives for sport withdrawal, a number of measurement concerns face the youth sport attrition researcher (Gould, 1983). These include the need to develop valid and reliable measures of achievement orientations and motives for withdrawal. In addition, methods of overcoming problems associated with giving socially desirable responses are needed. In the Petlichkoff (1982) study on high school dropouts, for instance, some of the former athletes indicated that injury was the major motive underlying the decision to discontinue. In some cases, however, further probing by the interviewer revealed that injury was used as a socially accepted reason, with the true reason for discontinuing (e.g., not as good as wanted to be) not initially cited. The social desirability problem can be overcome by using multiple assessment techniques (both self-report scales that make quantitative assessments and in-depth qualitative interviews where investigators can probe for additional responses) or designs where psychological data are collected before the season and prior to the decision to discontinue.

## Practical Implications for Preventing Attrition in Young Athletes

Although additional and improved research is needed, this does not imply that lack of practical implications characterizes the existing youth sport attrition research. In contrast, the existing research as summarized in this model has a number of important implications for those directly involved in children's sport.

A number of varied explanations exist for the high rate of attrition in youth sports. Some investigators have suggested that the high rate of attrition reflects a normal trial-and-error sampling process, in which children identify those activities they like best. Other reviewers contend that the high attrition rate results from inappropriate coaching and emotional stress. Neither of these views seems totally correct. Conflict of interest or interest in alternative activities was clearly the motive cited most often for discontinuing. Moreover, many children were found to leave one sport only to enter another. Some normal trial-and-error sport sampling is therefore occurring. At the same time, a substantial minority (15 to 20%) of young athletes discontinue because of more negative, adult-controlled motives such as an overemphasis on competition, lack of playing time, and excessive competitive stress. This supports the view that adult-controlled factors are related to attrition patterns in young athletes. Additionally, recent evidence reveals that various psychological constructs, such as low perceived ability, may underlie the change of interest in some children. An important implication of the research, then, is that trial-and-error sport sampling occurs on the part of some young athletes, whereas some children leave because of low perceived competence, lack of skill improvement, little fun, and an overly competitive environment (see Component 4 of Figure 2).

A second important implication resulting from the model focuses on the finding that children have multiple motives for participating in sports and in turn for discontinuing involvement. Major participation motives include developing skill, experiencing fun and excitement, achieving success, and being with friends. When these motives are not achieved, children weigh the costs versus benefits of participation (Component 3) and often withdraw citing other things to do as the reason. Knowing this, Gould and Horn (1984) have suggested that adult leaders structure the athletic environment so that these motives are fulfilled. Special emphasis should be placed on skill instruction for children of all ability levels. Excitement and fun must be maintained in practices and competitions by keeping young athletes active and by allowing all children the opportunity to participate. Special efforts should be made to meet the affiliation needs of young athletes. Finally, success should be more broadly defined as personal improvement, in contrast to competitive outcome.

A third implication generated from the model is that perceived competence and ability play important roles in the youth sport attrition process (see Component 4b). The development of perceived competence is influenced by the child's history of successes and failures at the activity (see the chapters by Horn and Weiss in this volume). Efforts must be made to develop realistic but positive perceptions of competence in young athletes. This can be accomplished by (a) equalizing competitive settings so that all children will experience some success, (b) providing positive but contingent evaluative feedback, (c) enhancing skill development, and (d) emphasizing the attainment of individual performance goals. Coaches working directly with young athletes must implement these procedures, as should additional significant others such as parents (Gould, in press).

## SUMMARY

The high rate of attrition in children's sport programs is one of the most significant issues facing those involved in youth sports. Fortunately, pediatric behavioral scientists have begun to study the area. The results of these investigations have shown that the attrition process is complex and is influenced by a variety of personal and situational variables. In particular, descriptive studies have revealed that conflicting and changing interests are the most often cited motives for youth sport withdrawal, with adult-controlled negative factors being cited by a much smaller but significant number of former athletes. The more recent theoretical literature supports these findings but also shows that various psychological constructs such as perceived competence, achievement orientations, and stress may at times underlie these changes in interest. A theoretical model of youth sport withdrawal integrating the descriptive findings in the area with initial theoretical explanations has been derived from this research. This model serves as both a guide for future research and as a means of organizing existing knowledge for practical application.

# Notes

1. An estimation of the number of children who participate in organized competitive sport throughout the world is difficult because few participation statistics are available. The few participation statistics available, however, do show a high rate of participation. In Australia, for example, Norman (1975) found that 48% of the children between 12 and 17 years old participated in sport, whereas estimates in the United States (Martens, 1978; Sapp & Haubenstricker, 1978) range from 35 to 40%. Because of the lower per capita income, decreased availability of leisure time, and lack of facilities in many Third World countries, youth sport participation probably does not approach the high rates found in western industrialized countries. Therefore,

a conservative rate of 20% of the world population of children between the ages of 5 and 14 years (United Nations, 1982) was used in making these estimates.

2. The respondents in this study were allowed to indicate more than one reason for their withdrawal. Hence, the percentage of responses exceeds 100%.

*Acknowledgments*

The author would like to thank Tony Byrne, Robert Levin, Rainer Martens, Linda Petlichkoff, and Maureen Weiss for their helpful comments during the development of this manuscript.

## REFERENCES

Burton, D., & Martens, R. (1986). Pinned by their goals: An exploratory investigation into why kids drop out of wrestling. *Journal of Sport Psychology, 8*(3), 183–197.

Ewing, M.E. (1981). *Achievement orientations and sport behavior of males and females*. Unpublished doctoral dissertation, University of Illinois, Urbana.

Feigley, D.A. (1984). Psychological burnout in high-level athletes. *The Physician and Sportsmedicine, 12*(10), 108–119.

Feltz, D.L., Gould, D., Horn, T.S., & Weiss, M.R. (1982, June). *Perceived competence among youth swimmers and dropouts*. Paper presented at the meeting of the North American Society for the Psychology of Sport and Physical Activity, College Park, MD.

Feltz, D.L., & Petlichkoff, L. (1983). Perceived competence among interscholastic sport participants and dropouts. *Canadian Journal of Applied Sport Science, 8*(4), 231–235.

Fry, D.A.P., McClements, J.D., & Sefton, J.M. (1981). *A report on participation in the Saskatoon Hockey Association*. Saskatoon, Canada: SASK Sport.

Gould, D. (1983). Future directions in youth sports participation motivation research. In L. Wankel & R. Wilberg (Eds.), *Psychology of sport and motor behavior: Research and practice* (pp. 137–145). Edmonton: University of Alberta, Faculty of Physical Education and Recreation.

Gould, D. (in press). Promoting positive sport experiences for children. In M.J. Ash & J. May (Eds.), *Sport psychology: The psychological health of the athlete*. Jamaca, NY: SP Medical and Scientific Books.

Gould, D., Feltz, D., Horn, T., & Weiss, M.R. (1982). Reasons for discontinuing involvement in competitive youth swimming. *Journal of Sport Behavior,* **5**, 155–165.

Gould, D., & Horn, T. (1984). Participation motivation in young athletes. In J.M. Silva & R.S. Weinberg (Eds.), *Psychological foundations of sport* (pp. 359–370). Champaign, IL: Human Kinetics.

Harter, S. (1978). Effectance motivation reconsidered: Toward a developmental model. *Human Development,* **21**, 34–64.

Harter, S.P. (1979). *Perceived competence scale for children.* (Manual: Form O). Denver, CO: University of Denver.

Harter, S. (1981). The development of competence motivation in the mastery of cognitive and physical skills: Is there still a place for joy? In G.C. Roberts & D.M. Landers (Eds.), *Psychology of motor behavior and sport—1980* (pp. 3–29). Champaign, IL: Human Kinetics.

Klint, K., & Weiss, M.R. (1986). Dropping in and dropping out: Participation motives of current and former youth gymnasts. *Canadian Journal of Applied Sport Sciences,* **11**(2), 106–114.

Lewin, K. (1935). *A dynamic theory of personality.* New York: McGraw-Hill.

Maehr, M.L., & Nicholls, J.G. (1980). Culture and achievement motivation: A second look. In N. Warren (Ed.), *Studies in cross-cultural psychology* (pp. 221–267). New York: Academic Press.

Martens, R. (1978). *Joy and sadness in children's sport.* Champaign, IL: Human Kinetics.

Martens, R. (1986). Youth sport in the USA. In M.R. Weiss & D. Gould (Eds.), *Sport for children and youths* (pp. 27–33). Champaign, IL: Human Kinetics.

Martens, R., & Seefeldt, V. (Eds.). (1979). *Guidelines in children's sports.* Washington, DC: American Alliance for Health, Physical Education, and Recreation.

McPherson, B.D., Guppy, L.N., & McKay, J.P. (1976). The social structure of the game and sport milieu. In J.G. Albinson & G.M. Andrews (Eds.), *Children in sport and physical activity* (pp. 161–200). Baltimore, MD: University Park.

Nettleton, B. (1979, June). *The social institution of sport today and tomorrow.* Paper presented at the "Sport Today: Health or Disability" seminar, Lincoln Institute of Health Sciences, Melbourne, Australia.

Norman, M.J. (1975). *Youth say report: The recreational priorities of Australian young people.* Canberra: Australian Government Publishing Service.

Ogilvie, B.C., & Howe, M.A. (1982). Career crisis in sport. In T. Orlick, J.T. Partington, & J.H. Salmela (Eds.), *Mental training for coaches and athletes* (pp. 176–183). Ottawa, Canada: Coaching Association of Canada.

Orlick, T.D. (1973, January/February). Children's sport—A revolution is coming. *Canadian Association for Health, Physical Education and Recreation Journal*, pp. 12–14.

Orlick, T.D. (1974, November/December). The athletic dropout—A high price of inefficiency. *Canadian Association for Health, Physical Education and Recreation Journal*, pp. 21–27.

Orlick, T.D., & Botterill, C. (1975). *Every kid can win*. Chicago, IL: Nelson-Hall.

Petlichkoff, L.M. (1982). *Motives interscholastic athletes have for participation and reasons for discontinued involvement in school sponsored sport*. Unpublished master's thesis, Michigan State University, East Lansing.

Pooley, J.C. (1981). *Drop-outs from sport: A case study for boys age-group soccer*. Paper presented at the meeting of the American Alliance for Health, Physical Education, Recreation, and Dance, Boston, MA.

Roberts, G.C. (1984). Achievement motivation in children's sport. *Advances in Motivation and Achievement, 3*, 251–281.

Roberts, G.C., Kleiber, D.A., & Duda, J.L. (1981). An analysis of motivation in children's sport: The role of perceived competence in participation. *Journal of Sport Psychology, 3*, 203–211.

Robertson, I. (1981, January). *Children's perceived satisfactions and stresses in sport*. Paper presented at the Australian Conference on Health, Physical Education and Recreation Biennial Conference, Melbourne.

Robinson, T., & Carron, A. (1982). Personal and situational factors associated with dropping out versus maintaining participation in competitive sport. *Journal of Sport Psychology, 4*, 364–378.

Sapp, M., & Haubenstricker, J. (1978). *Motivation for joining and reasons for not continuing in youth sport programs in Michigan*. Paper presented at the meeting of the American Alliance for Health, Physical Education, Recreation, and Dance, Kansas City, MO.

Sefton, J.M.M., & Fry, D.A.P. (1981). *A report on participation in competitive swimming*. Saskatoon, Canada: Canadian Amateur Swimming Association (Saskatchewan Section).

Smith, R.E. (1986). Toward a cognitive-affective model of athletic burnout. *Journal of Sport Psychology, 8*, 36–50.

Smith, R.E., Smoll, F.L., Hunt, E., Curtis, B., & Coppel, D.B. (1979). Psychology and the bad news bears. In G.C. Roberts & K.M. Newell (Eds.),

*Psychology of motor behavior and sport—1978* (pp. 109-130). Champaign, IL: Human Kinetics.

Thibaut, J.W., & Kelly, H.H. (1959). *The social psychology of groups*. New York: Wiley.

United Nations. (1982). *United Nations 1982 demographic yearbook*. New York: United Nations Publications.

Weiss, M.R., Bredemeier, B.J., & Shewchuk, R.M. (1986). The dynamics of perceived competence, perceived control, and motivation orientation in youth sport. In M.R. Weiss & D. Gould (Eds.), *Sport for children and youths* (pp. 89-102). Champaign, IL: Human Kinetics.

White, R.W. (1959). Motivation reconsidered: The concept of competence. *Psychological Review,* **66**, 297-333.

# 5

# Self-Esteem and Achievement in Children's Sport and Physical Activity

**Maureen R. Weiss**

The topic that seems to stir the most attention in the social psychological literature on children's sport is simply the "self." Various forms of hyphenated constructs such as self-concept, self-esteem, self-confidence, self-image, and self-worth abound in texts and scholarly articles that preach the beneficial outcomes of participating in sport and physical activity. The majority of texts on elementary physical education and youth sports states that improvement in physical skills and encouragement for mastery attempts will undoubtedly result in enhanced self-esteem on the part of the recipients (see Kirchner, 1985; Morris & Stiehl, 1985). Despite these claims of heightened self-evaluations resulting from physical competence, little substantive evidence exists to support them.

The self-concept has been a central construct in education for years. Self-concept has traditionally referred to the descriptions or labels that an individual attaches to him- or herself, such as physical attributes, behavioral character-istics, or emotional qualities (e.g., "happy with the way I am"). Self-esteem represents the evaluative and affective component of one's self-concept; that is, it refers to the qualitative judgments and feelings attached to the description one assigns to self. In many cases, these terms are used interchangeably (Shavelson, Hubner, & Stanton, 1976; Wells & Marwell, 1976) because evaluation and affect appear to be natural consequences of self-description. In this chapter, the terms self-concept and self-esteem will be used interchangeably and will encompass the description of, evaluation of, and affect toward competencies in domain-specific areas. Coopersmith's (1967) definition of self-esteem has been one of the most popular and most relevant for application to the physical domain. According to Coopersmith, self-esteem is:

> the evaluation which the individual makes and customarily maintains with regard to him-self: It expresses an attitude of approval or disapproval and indicates the extent to which an individual believes himself to be capable, significant, successful and worthy. In short, self-esteem is a personal judgment of worthiness that is expressed in the attitudes the individual conveys to others by verbal reports and other expressive behavior. (p. 5)

Self-esteem continues to be a primary focus in educational contexts because it is considered to be a major factor influencing such processes as motivation, persistence, standards of success, and causal attributions for success and failure outcomes. Given the importance attached to a positive self-esteem in physical education and sport, substantial research might have long ago established the connection between gains in physical competence and feelings of self-worth. However, the lack of a guiding theoretical perspective has precluded major advances in understanding this relationship. Adopting a theoretical approach to self-esteem would provide a parsimonious and practical approach to effecting self-esteem change in sport environments.

A theoretical approach—and, more importantly, one that employs the use of cognitive-developmental criteria—is critical for understanding how self-esteem is formed, factors that mediate the self-esteem/performance relationship, and ways in which positive changes can be promoted. In essence, such a theoretical approach utilizes knowledge about the nature of developmental changes in the ways children judge and evaluate their capabilities and ultimately describes, explains, and predicts the relationship between level of self-esteem and partici-pation behavior in the physical domain (Weiss & Bredemeier, 1983). Merely employing a pretest/posttest research design of the effects of participation on self-esteem is not as revealing as identifying how the "self" develops and designing programs to facilitate increases in self-esteem.

The purpose of this chapter will be to review the development of self-esteem within a theoretical framework, the notion of domain-specific self-esteems, the relationship between self-esteem and physical achievement, and the means by which practitioners can implement knowledge about self-esteem to physical activity settings.

## THE DEVELOPMENT OF SELF-ESTEEM

Given the definition of self-esteem as the extent to which the child evaluates him- or herself to be competent, successful, and worthy, the first critical question to understanding self-esteem is, How are these evaluations formed? A number of theories have emerged to explain the development of self-esteem as well as the major characteristics that distinguish its role in behavioral processes. A brief description of the major theories will provide a useful foundation for understanding self-esteem development, followed by a consideration of the commonalities among these major self theories.

### Major Theories of Self-Esteem Development

William James (1890) was responsible for establishing the foundation on which all modern theories of the self have been based. James explicitly addressed the meaning of self-esteem in relation to actual achievement. Specifically, he stated that a person's feelings of worth are determined by the ratio of one's actual accomplishments to one's aspirations. The affect resulting from such evaluations was an important element of self-esteem for James.

In contrast to James's emphasis on competence and the affect associated with its evaluation, Cooley (1902/1956) focused on the central role that social interactions play in the development of the self. He described the role of significant others in self-concept development as a social mirror, one that the child uses to imagine what others think of his or her appearance, motives, and behaviors. He stated that children actively formulate their own sense of self-worth by associating a self-evaluation with the judgment they think others ascribe to their behavior. Cooley subsumed these ideas under the metaphor of reflected or *looking-glass self:* "Each to each a looking glass/Reflects the other that doth pass" (pp. 183–184). This approach is often called *symbolic interactionism* and refers to children's understanding of how their behavior affects others' behavior and that others' behavior is a reflection of themselves.

Mead (1934) elaborated upon Cooley's ideas of the self as emerging through social interactions. The critical feature in Mead's theory of the development of self is the child's cognitive activity in interpreting him- or herself relative to the social milieu. This contrasted with Cooley's emphasis on the affective component. Mead implied that the child observes significant others and takes the attitude that others take toward him or her. He called this behavior taking the role of the *generalized other*, and it includes the ability of perspective taking. Interestingly, Mead highlighted the importance of play and games as contributing factors in the evaluation of the self-concept as children become engaged in role playing.

Combs and Snygg (1959) viewed self-esteem from a perceptual or phenomenological perspective that emphasizes the various perceptions or conscious awareness that individuals regard as characteristic of themselves. The individual's unique collection of self-referent concepts is thought to be a product of one's perceived experiences relative to the satisfaction of needs for feelings of adequacy and acceptance. Changes in the self-concept, according to this position, occur when the individual faces experiences that are not congruent with one's self-perceptions. In this case, the individual attempts to preserve one's self-ideas and feelings of adequacy and self-worth. The dynamics underlying the phenomenal view of the self carry particular significance for sport practitioners, which will be addressed later.

Rosenberg (1979) has come closest to addressing self-esteem from a cognitive-developmental theoretical perspective. He found that there were developmental changes in how children and adolescents described themselves. Whereas young children (about age 8) made self-descriptions based on concrete, observable characteristics such as physical attributes and material possessions, children in the later elementary ages emphasized trait-like characteristics, such as being nice and friendly. In adolescence (about age 14), individuals tended to use more abstract self-definitions based on psychological processes such as inner thoughts, emotions, attitudes, and motives. Thus, Rosenberg proposed that both structure and content change with regard to self-esteem development.

The theories of self presented above do not exhaust all theories. Instead, major theories that appear to hold the most support or acceptance among psychologists as well as having particular relevance for physical activity and sport settings have been described here. In addition, these theories taken together provide common principles regarding development of the self. These principles are discussed next.

## Common Themes of Self-Esteem Theories

*Self-esteem is a product of social interactions.* The sources for self-esteem development rest primarily in reflected appraisals (looking-glass self) and social comparisons. Reflected appraisals refer to those direct and indirect communications from significant others regarding approval or disapproval of the child's behaviors and performances. Factors such as the credibility of the appraiser, discrepancy between the appraisal and one's own self-views, and number and consistency of appraisals all influence their acceptance or rejection by the individual, as well as their effect on self-esteem. Recently, Coakley (1984) stated that "the physical act of involvement in sport experiences is insignificant in light of the structure and dynamics of the relationships encountered by involvement. Involvement itself takes on meaning through relationships with others" (p. 2).

The other major source of self-esteem garnered through social interactions is social comparison. Children compare their competencies to those of their peers in order to discern their level of competence and worth in the physical domain. Social comparison processes are especially salient when discussing sport and physical activity because competition by nature entails the comparison of one's skills to others (Scanlan, 1982). Recent research indicates that social comparison is a developmental phenomenon, with children beginning to engage in comparison at about age 6 or 7 (Ruble, Boggiano, Feldman, & Loebl, 1980) and intensifying during the fourth or fifth grades (Scanlan, 1982).

*Self-esteem is multidimensional in nature.* A second common element to most theories of self-esteem is that there are multiple "selves," suggesting that self-evaluation and affect depend upon the domain serving as the reference for one's judgments. For example, a person's self-esteem in the physical domain may be high, but evaluations of competence in relating with peers may be low. In addition to the notion of multiple selves, many self theorists have cast self-esteem into a hierarchy of dimensions (Coopersmith, 1967; Epstein, 1973; Harter, 1983; Shavelson, Hubner, & Stanton, 1976). Specifically, a global self-esteem (independent of a competence domain) tops the hierarchy, under which several specific dimensions of self are contained. Coopersmith (1967), Epstein (1973), and Harter (1983) all delineated four dimensions underlying global self-esteem:

- competence, or success in meeting achievement demands

- social acceptance, or attention, worthiness, and positive reinforcement received from significant others

- control, or feelings of internal responsibility for outcomes

- virtue, or adherence to moral and ethical standards

In addition to the four dimensions subsumed under global self-esteem, each of these dimensions can be divided further into situational specific categories. For example, competence can be split into cognitive, social, and physical sub-areas, and social acceptance can include peers and adults. The notion of global self-esteem as well as the more differentiated view of the self have not only found a place in most recent scale-construction efforts by researchers but appear to offer an appealing framework in which a developmental theory of self-esteem can be established.

*Affect is a central aspect in the development of self-esteem.* Affect is considered to be central in formulations of self-esteem (Cooley, 1902/1956; Harter, 1981a; James, 1890; Rosenberg, 1979). In particular, the pride and joy or shame and disappointment that accompany perceptions of competence or incompetence are thought to influence future motivated behavior powerfully.

This aspect of self-esteem development is especially noteworthy in light of developments in the area of attribution theory. When successful performance outcomes are attributed to internal factors such as ability and effort, positive affect results. When unsuccessful outcomes are attributed to internal factors, most notably a lack of ability, negative affect results. The importance of affect as it pertains to attribution lies in its predictable effect on future motivated behavior (Diener & Dweck, 1978; Dweck & Elliott, 1984). For example, Diener and Dweck (1978) found that children who attributed mistakes to lack of ability expressed negative affect toward the task and no longer wanted to participate.

Sport scientists and practitioners are often reluctant to consider the role of affect or emotions in motivated behavior or performance outcome. However, recent attempts to incorporate both positive and negative affect into models of sport-related behavior (Harter, 1981b; Passer, 1984; Scanlan & Lewthwaite, 1984, 1986; Vallerand, 1983) may stimulate others to arouse this all-important construct as it relates to self-esteem. Harter (1981a) implores that "affect should be given center stage" when considering the study of motivated behavior (p. 5).

*The salience of an activity to an individual will determine the degree to which success or failure affects one's self-esteem.* Coined by Rosenberg (1979) as "psychological centrality," the importance that an individual attaches to a particular domain or activity will determine the extent to which a successful or unsuccessful outcome will affect the individual's self-esteem. For example, a child's low perceived competence in physical skills may not have a negative effect on total self-esteem because he or she does not value physical competence as important for being successful.

Rosenberg (1979) notes that components of the self-concept are of unequal centrality to the individual's concerns. The importance of a specific self-esteem component to the individual is highly related to the individual's overall evaluations of self-worth. As an illustration, Rosenberg describes four boys, all with a favorable global self-esteem but each stemming from separate judgmental criteria—academics, athletics, physical appearance, and music. "Thus, the individual strives to excel at that which he values and to value that at which he excels" (Rosenberg, 1979, p. 75).

The construct of salience of a particular achievement domain has particular relevance in understanding the self-esteem of children and adolescents in physical activity settings. All too often, the importance of a particular activity to an individual has been neglected, with success and failure outcomes assumed to influence all individuals equally. However, unsuccessful outcomes in an area not deemed salient by a young child should not be detrimental to his or her self-esteem. Conversely, where sport competence is salient in the lives of most boys (Coleman, 1961; Eitzen, 1976), it is not surprising that anxiety has been found to be strongly linked to self-evaluation and performance outcomes (Scanlan & Passer, 1978; Shewchuk & Weiss, 1986). In contrast, where sport competence has not been as salient in the lives of young girls (Feltz, 1978; Williams & White, 1985), one would expect possible gender differences in affect and perceived competence as a result of performance outcomes.

*Self-esteem is viewed to have a motivational influence on behavior.* The basic motivational elements associated with self-esteem have been self-enhancement and self-maintenance. Self-enhancement emphasizes growth and expansion of one's self-esteem, whereas self-maintenance stresses the preservation of what one already has (Gecas, 1982). Lecky (1945) clarified his understanding of the motivational value of self-esteem by seeking a perceptual or phenomenological perspective. His self-consistency theory describes the notion that individuals behave and interpret experiences in ways that confirm their beliefs of themselves and preserve the integrity of their self-judgments. Experiences are thus interpreted as congruent with one's already established self-perceptions, and individuals will inevitably behave in a manner consistent with their self-view and reject evaluations or information that do not validate these perceptions.

The motivational value of self-esteem as a consistency motive is perhaps illuminated in terms of Bandura's (1977) self-efficacy theory. According to this theory, a person's expectation of producing the behaviors needed to be successful will determine the amount of effort and persistence displayed under adverse conditions. Individuals low in self-efficacy tend to avoid achievement situations and exert little effort and/or give up when the "going gets tough." Individuals with high efficacy expectations, conversely, try hard, persist under challenging situations, and eventually conquer the task. Thus, self-views can influence subsequent behavior substantially. Within a self-consistency stance, individuals behave in a manner consistent with their self-views so as to preserve their self-perceptions.

Given the need for individuals to maintain or enhance self-esteem, individuals may likely develop strategies for dealing with situations that threaten it. For example, Covington and Beery (1977) found that children with low self-esteem adopted strategies such as avoiding participation, not trying hard, and setting unrealistic goals to create a situation whereby they could preserve what little sense of self-worth they possessed. In terms of attribution theory, the child who experiences success in light of low self-esteem will likely ascribe the outcome to some capricious factor as opposed to personal causation. In essence, the child discounts information such as ability attributions for success that are not congruent with one's self-views of competence. Over time, low self-esteem children tend to adopt failure-prone strategies and attribute unsuccessful outcomes to lack of ability and successes to environmental causes beyond their control (Diener & Dweck, 1978; Dweck & Elliott, 1984; Martens, Christina, Sharkey, & Harvey, 1981).

## PERCEIVED COMPETENCE:
## THE NOTION OF DOMAIN-SPECIFIC SELF-ESTEEM

Addressing the construct of self-esteem is difficult without also considering the development of domain-specific skills. The dimension of competence has been an integral part in most theories of self-esteem and is delineated as a central dimension in several multidimensional models of the self (Epstein, 1973; Harter,

1983; Shavelson, Hubner, & Stanton, 1976). Thus, a child's perceptions of competence are a central construct in understanding self-esteem development and achievement motivation.

Harter (1978, 1981a, 1981b, 1983, 1985) has written extensively on the dimension of competence within the larger scope of general self-worth. She has described a theoretical framework for explaining how the dimension of competence undergoes developmental change, particularly regarding its impact on the structure of self-esteem. The dynamics of competence and its relation to self-esteem are subsumed under effectance or competence motivation theory, a theory originally expressed by White (1959).

White contended that individuals are motivated to have an effect on their environment and to engage in mastery attempts. When these attempts result in competent or successful performance, individuals experience intrinsic pleasure and, in turn, maintain or enhance their urge toward competence. White viewed behaviors such as curiosity, challenge, and play as examples whereby the child's urge toward competence was satisfied by positive affect. A notable shortcoming of White's theory is the absence of operational constructs (e.g., effectance, feelings of efficacy) and thus the inability to test the model empirically.

Harter and her colleagues (Connell, 1985; Harter, 1978, 1981a, 1981b, 1981c, 1983; Harter & Connell, 1982; Harter & Pike, 1983) have cast competence motivation theory into an empirically testable and practically useful model. The refined model is particularly attractive in its sensitivity to developmental changes and individual differences within developmental levels. Thus, steps toward a developmental and comprehensive theory of self-worth, differentiated into multiple dimensions, have been taken very carefully and successfully. A schematic of Harter's refinement of White's competence motivation theory can be seen in Figure 1.

Harter's (1978, 1981b) refinement and extension of White's original formulations opened the way for empirical testing by not only expanding the model to include several constructs known to be related to competence but also by providing operational definitions for these constructs. The development of valid and reliable scales to measure these constructs has been invaluable in contributing to investigators' ability to conduct empirical studies on self-esteem and competence motivation in children and adolescents.

Harter viewed competence motivation as a multidimensional motive responsive to the influence of several social and psychological factors. The components of the competence model are integrally related to the development of self-esteem and provide an appealing framework from which to study the patterns of self-esteem and achievement behavior in sport and physical activity. Finally, the model allows for an investigation of self-esteem from a developmental perspective, an approach neglected in the past but so critical in understanding children's psychosocial growth through sport (Weiss & Bredemeier, 1983).

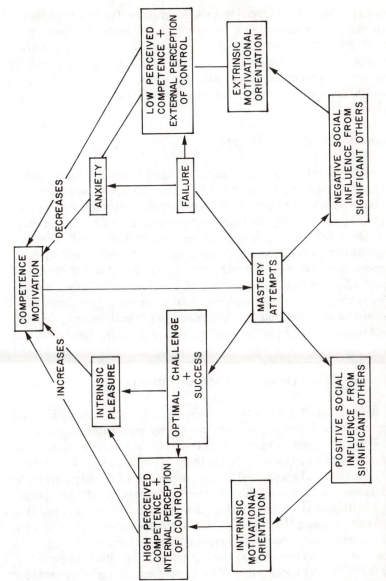

**Figure 1** Harter's version of White's competence motivation theory.

The components that are integral to the multidimensional model of competence (or effectance) motivation are (a) the notion of domain-specific mastery attempts, (b) the consequences of both success and failure experiences, (c) success based on optimal challenges, (d) influence from significant others, (e) intrinsic/extrinsic motivational orientation, (f) perceived competence, (g) perceived control, and (h) affective outcomes of mastery attempts. Descriptions of each component follow.

## Domain-Specific Mastery Attempts

Competence or effectance motivation (at the top of the model) refers to the child's urge to demonstrate abilities and affect his or her physical or social environment. Whereas White primarily viewed competence motivation from a somewhat global perspective by delineating the consequences of mastery attempts per se, Harter differentiated general competence into three specific domains: (a) cognitive (school performance), (b) social (peer relationships), and (c) physical (athletic prowess). This conceptualization is consonant with the notion of multiple "selves" in that individuals have different capabilities in these mastery domains and also different salience hierarchies. These two aspects, actual competence and the importance attached to success in a particular domain, considerably influence subsequent evaluations of one's competence and future motivated behavior.

## Success and Failure Outcomes of Mastery Attempts

Whereas White attended only to the antecedents and consequences of successful mastery outcomes, Harter's model takes into account the antecedents and consequences of both success and failure. The results of success are pictured to the left of the diagram and those of failure to the right. Successful outcomes of mastery attempts are hypothesized to result in positive affect and positive self-regard; failure, on the other hand, leads to anxiety and negative self-perceptions. Because of the inherent potential and opportunity to focus on mastery products in the various domains, Harter (1982a) underscores the necessity for redirecting our efforts at the level of the mastery process to become competent, manifested in such behaviors as choosing to participate, exerting effort, or persisting amidst the struggle of learning new skills. She suggests that reinforcement for mastery attempts collaborates with the child's own intrinsic desire to master and control the environment. Further, Harter states that "to the extent that we attend primarily to the product during the early years, and ignore those behavioral attempts which constitute the process of production, we may ultimately attenuate the child's desire to engage in the mastery process itself, and may weaken the child's sense of control over such efforts" (Harter, 1982a, p. 11). Significant others must make a more concerted effort to reward the mastery attempt itself as a worthwhile endeavor in order to ensure such positive consequences as intrinsic desire and joyful behavior.

## The Construct of Optimal Challenge

With respect to successful outcomes, Harter clarified the definition of success by adding optimal challenge as a requirement for maximized positive self-perceptions. Optimal challenge refers to tasks or situations in which the degree of difficulty is carefully matched to the learner's developmental capabilities. Harter (1974) has found that optimal challenges that are mastered result in the greatest amount of pleasure, as opposed to tasks that are too easy or even too difficult in relation to one's capabilities. Tasks that are too difficult result in frustration and anxiety, whereas those not challenging enough result in boredom and reduced motivation.

## Influence by Significant Others

In addition to self-perceptions, affect, and future motivated behavior being influenced by successful mastery attempts, the role of significant others such as parents, teachers, and peers plays a major part in the formation of these outcomes as well. Evaluation in the form of reinforcement and modeling of approval toward mastery attempts affects the competence and control dimensions of self-esteem, as well as the motivational orientation of the child. The extension of White's model to include this crucial socialization aspect is necessarily dictated by the consensus among theorists that self-esteem development is social in origin.

The combination of mastery attempts, the outcome of those attempts, and adult feedback for mastery strivings is a crucial aspect of Harter's model. When a significant adult conveys positive reinforcement for independent mastery attempts and demonstrates approval for these attempts to the child, enhancement of intrinsic motives (mastery goals) and perceptions of competence and control result. When the child's mastery attempts are not rewarded or approved by important others, the need for extrinsic incentives increases, along with perceptions of incompetence and external perceptions of control. Over time, the outcomes of significant other influences may either stimulate or attenuate future competence motivation.

The developmental nature of the theory is highlighted here in that younger children (ages 8 to 11) tend to rate evaluative feedback from parents as a more important source of information about their competence than do older children (ages 12 to 14), whereas older children rate social comparison sources more important than younger children (Horn & Hasbrook, 1986). Additionally, younger children rely more on game outcome (winning/losing) as a source of competence judgments than do older children (Horn & Hasbrook, 1986), suggesting that developmental differences exist in how children judge qualitative and quantitative aspects of their performance.

## Intrinsic/Extrinsic Motivational Orientation

The construct of motivational orientation refers to the motivational stance adopted by the child toward a specific achievement domain and provides a measure of the underlying reasons for engaging in particular achievement-related behaviors. The major question addressed by motivational orientation is, To what degree is a child's motivation for learning determined by her or his intrinsic interest in learning and mastery, curiosity, and preference for challenge, in contrast to a more extrinsic orientation in which the child is motivated to obtain teacher approval and/or grades and is dependent on the teacher for guidance? Harter (1981c) formulated a valid and reliable scale to measure motivational orientation in the classroom. She found developmental trends with respect to components of motivational orientation: A shift from intrinsic to extrinsic orientation occurred from Grades 3 to 9 on preference for challenge, curiosity, and mastery, but an opposite shift took place, from extrinsic to intrinsic, on preference for independent judgment and use of internal criteria to judge performance.

## Perceived Competence

The construct of perceived competence is a central one in Harter's model and the one most pertinent to our discussion of self-esteem and achievement. Perceived competence refers to one's domain-specific self-esteem as it relates to the competence dimension of self-esteem. Harter delineated perceived competence in the cognitive, social, and physical realms, as well as retaining a measure of general self-worth. Because various measures of general and domain-specific self-esteem have been fraught with problems (Wylie, 1979), Harter (1982b) devised the Perceived Competence Scale for Children, with consistent and adequate reliability and validity characteristics for children from Grades 3 through 9. Harter and Pike (1983) later extended this scale to pictorial versions appropriate for preschool-kindergarten and first-second grades.

The developmental nature of competence motivation theory emerges again upon examination of the perceived competence construct. Harter (1982b) found that children in Grades 3 through 9 clearly made distinctions between competence domains in the cognitive, social, and physical realms. However, Harter and Pike (1983) found that 4- to 7-year-old children did not differentiate competence domains as clearly. Children viewed cognitive and physical competence as similar from the overall standpoint that kids either did well at things or did not do well. A second group of items was defined by peer social acceptance and acceptance by mother. Thus, for children in preschool through second grade, general competence and social acceptance appear to be the salient self-esteem constructs, whereas perceived social, cognitive, and physical competence and general self-worth are all deemed distinct by third through ninth graders.

## Perceived Control

The construct of perceived control is a measure of the child's understanding of who or what is responsible for behavioral outcomes in each of the three competence domains. The construct of control was another dimension of self-esteem identified earlier and one that closely parallels perceived competence in Harter's model. Measures of the child's perceptions of his or her influence over environmental events, along with perceived competence, are also thought to impact significantly on motivated behavior and actual achievement. Interestingly, Connell's (1980) investigations of children's perceptions of control led him to three independent sources of control: internal, powerful others, and unknown. The internal and powerful others (or external) dimensions have been employed in previous scales (Nowicki & Strickland, 1973) but the unknown scale had not been previously encountered. In essence, Connell found that children sometimes indicated that they simply did not know who or what was responsible for their successes and failures and thus established a pertinent dimension in the assessment of perceived control.

From a developmental perspective, younger children are most likely to indicate a lack of understanding over what caused successful or unsuccessful outcomes. With age, children begin to identify either internal (e.g., ability, effort) or external factors (e.g., luck, task difficulty), depending on the quality of adult feedback in response to mastery attempts and one's motivational orientation.

According to Harter's model, perceptions of competence and control are both primarily influenced by performance outcomes, significant other reactions to mastery attempts and outcomes, and motivational orientation. Thus, game outcome, coaching style, and parental and/or peer reactions to a child's performance attempts can be salient sources of self-esteem development in the physical domain. Because children differ developmentally in the sources of information most salient for their competence judgments, the need exists for careful instructional strategies and explanations for successful and unsuccessful outcomes in sport.

## Affective Outcomes of Achievement Strivings: Enjoyment and Anxiety

Little attention has been afforded the role of affect in self-esteem development despite the historical precedence of James and Cooley in emphasizing its importance. Harter (1981a) contends that engaging in mastery behavior results in joy and pleasure when the individual is successful and in anxiety when unsuccessful. These affective reactions in turn have implications for future motivated behavior in similar achievement situations in the form of choice of activities, effort, and persistence. Interestingly, in a statement linking the relationship among affect, perceived competence, motivational orientation, and perceived control in the cognitive versus the physical domain, Harter (1981a) concludes:

> The picture looks somewhat less bleak in the area of sports. As adults, we have yet to inter-fere to the same degree. While an evaluative aura exists, sports are much more under the control of peer influence. Intrinsic interest in sports is much higher than in school, and success per se is viewed as less important. Performance anxiety is much lower in the athletic domain, compared to scholastic achievement. Children often link their sense of physical competence to their ability to master the skills of a sport and to their enjoyment of the activity, in contrast to the cognitive domain where the evaluation of adult authority figures and the speed of their performance are major determinants of their perceived competence. Efficacy pleasure is at least alive in the domain of sports, but is it well? (p. 27)

Some, perhaps many, sport scientists and practitioners might take issue with such statements as ''under the control of peer influence'' or ''success per se is viewed as less important.'' Certainly, numerous studies examining the existence of anxiety in youth sports (Gould, Horn, & Spreeman, 1983; Scanlan & Lewthwaite, 1984; Scanlan & Passer, 1978, 1979) have established a pervasive relationship between social evaluation potential and anxiety in sport. The incidence of positive affect is less understood, although recent studies (Scanlan & Lewthwaite, 1986; Wankel & Kreisel, 1985) have begun to explore enjoyment factors in youth sports.

To summarize, Harter's model of competence motivation has been carefully conceived with special attention to the role of developmental, cognitive, affective, and motivational factors. Her focus on self-esteem from a multifactor approach within a developmental perspective provides an excellent research model from which sport scientists can test hypotheses in the physical domain. Weiss and Bredemeier (1983) have recently provided guidelines for stimulating empirical verification of Harter's theory in the physical domain. However, despite the appeal and apparent generalizability of Harter's competence motivation theory to youth sports, relatively little research has been initiated to test the validity of her model in the sport setting. Those studies that have been conducted, however, reveal exceptional promise of competence motivation theory as a comprehensive framework for understanding children's perceived competence (self-esteem) and achievement in sport and physical activity.

## Sport-Specific Studies of Competence Motivation

Four studies have examined children's participation motives from the standpoint of competence motivation theory (Feltz & Petlichkoff, 1983; Klint, 1985; Klint & Weiss, in press; Roberts, Kleiber, & Duda, 1981). Roberts et al. (1981) found that participants can be distinguished from nonparticipants in youth sport by a number of achievement-related characteristics. Specifically, participants scored higher in perceived physical competence, had higher success expectancies, and were more likely to attribute successful outcomes to ability than nonparticipants. The authors concluded that their results support the notion that perceived competence not only appears to influence achievement-related behaviors but also may be a deciding factor affecting children's participatory patterns in sport.

In a study comparing current and former junior and senior high school athletes, Feltz and Petlichkoff (1983) found that current participants scored higher in perceived physical competence than did ex-athletes. The authors suggested, in accordance with Harter's theory, that when individuals no longer perceive themselves as competent in sports, they will likely discontinue participation in that particular sport.

These findings were not supported by Klint (1985) in her investigation of the motives and self-perceptions of recreational and currently and formerly competitive youth gymnasts. Results revealed that whereas former and recreational gymnasts scored higher on perceived social competence than did current gymnasts, the former and current gymnasts did not differ in perceived physical competence. Although these results were contrary to those reported earlier, they are explainable when considering the transitory nature of "participant status" of young athletes; that is, children and youth appear to be nonparticipants, participants, and former participants (no longer involved in a particular sport) at various phases of their life. Thus, the nature of participant status must be accurately defined when examining self-perceptions of youth sport participants.

The difficulties associated with defining participant status prompted Klint and Weiss (in press) to examine the relationship between perceptions of competence and particular motives for sport participation. Children who were current members of youth gymnastic programs were categorized as high or low in perceived competence and were compared on specific motives for participating in youth sports. Results partially supported the notions of competence motivation theory in demonstrating that perceived competence and particular participant motives were related. Specifically, those who were high in perceived physical competence rated skill development reasons as more important for their participation than those low in perceived competence. In addition, those high in perceived social competence were more motivated into sport roles by affiliation-related aspects of involvement such as group atmosphere and being with friends. In sum, Harter's theory of competence motivation appears to offer a great deal of promise in understanding the relationship between self-esteem and participation motivation.

In addition to the role of perceived competence in understanding participatory behaviors, Harter's model highlights the importance that significant others' feedback and attained skill level impart on competence perceptions. Horn (1985) was interested in examining the influence of coaches' behavior in response to desirable and undesirable performance on junior high school athletes' perceptions of competence and control. Coaches' behaviors over a number of practices and games were recorded and perceptions of competence and control were assessed during the pre- and postseason using Harter's (1982b) and Connell's (1980) measures of these respective constructs. Results revealed that although attained skill level accounted for the most variance in players' psychosocial growth over the season, the coaches' use of reinforcement, nonreinforcement, and punishment was also important in explaining changes in perceived competence.

Scale construction efforts to test the applicability of Harter's measures in the cognitive domain to the sport domain have been successful (Ulrich, in press; Weiss, Bredemeier, & Shewchuk, 1985; Weiss & Shewchuk, 1985). Ulrich built upon the Pictorial Scale of Perceived Competence and Social Acceptance for Young Children (Harter & Pike, 1983) by including depictions of fundamental motor skills (e.g., throwing, catching) and motor abilities (e.g., strength) to which young children in physical education could relate. She found that these items, when added to those in Harter and Pike's original scale, contributed to a higher internal consistency of the scale items. Weiss et al. (1985) conducted a confirmatory factor analysis to test the fit of Harter's model for motivational orientation in the classroom to data collected on items modified for assessing motivational orientation in the sport setting. Results revealed an overall adequate fit of the model to the data although some differences in subscale items were found. In a subsequent study, Weiss and Shewchuk (1985) replicated and validated these findings. Thus, a motivational orientation in sport scale has been identified for use in the study of competence motivation in sport.

Little information exists about the processes children use to form perceptions of competence. Horn and Hasbrook (1986) were particularly interested in what sources of competence information children use, specifically in relation to developmental and gender differences. They administered an adaptation of Minton's (1979) Competence Information Scale to 273 children ranging in age from 8 to 14 years. The information sources to which children were asked to rate importance in judging their competence clustered into six factors: social comparison; social evaluation (parents, spectators); social evaluation (coaches, peers, spectators); internal sources; game outcome; and affect. More importantly, Horn and Hasbrook found that the saliency of these information sources varied by developmental level. Specifically, they found that the oldest age group, 12- to 14-year-olds, rated social comparison information sources significantly higher in importance than did the 8- to 9-year-olds or the 10- to 11-year-olds. Further, the two younger age groups rated outcome and social evaluation from parents and spectators as more important sources of information than did the oldest group. These results provided tremendous insight into the qualitative changes that occur when children of various ages evaluate their competence in the physical domain.

In a similar vein, Horn and Weiss (1986) were interested in developmental differences in children's ability to assess their achievement competencies accurately.

The researchers hypothesized that accuracy of self-perceptions occur with age and that they may be due to changes in the criteria children use to assess their competence. Children ($N = 134$) ranging in age from 8 to 13 years were administered questionnaires to assess their perceptions of physical competence and the criteria they use to evaluate their competence. Corresponding measures of the children's actual competence were obtained via performance measures and teachers' skill ratings. The hypotheses were supported in that children's perceptions of their physical competence in relation to actual measures became more accurate with age. Additionally, dependence on social evaluation declined with age, whereas orientation toward peer comparison increased as a means to assess personal competencies. These results were consistent with Horn and Hasbrook (1986) and emphasized the developmental nature of Harter's theory.

Finally, Weiss, Bredemeier, and Shewchuk (1986) used causal modeling procedures in examining the directional relationships among perceived competence, perceived control, physical achievement, and motivational orientation in 155 children aged 8 to 12 who were participating in a summer sport camp. The results showed that perceptions of one's competence in sport causally influenced physical achievement and motivational orientation. Further, perceived control was found to influence achievement and motivational orientation, indicating that the child who understands the causes of successful or unsuccessful outcomes experiences higher achievement and an intrinsic motivational orientation.

In summary, Harter's (1978, 1981b) competence motivation theory, with its multidimensional and comprehensive perspective of the development of self-perceptions, offers a relevant, appealing theoretical framework for understanding children's self-esteem development and achievement in sport. The few studies that have been conducted to verify the generalizability of Harter's theory have found constructs pertinent in her model also salient to physical activity settings. The opportunities for continued research from a competence motivation theoretical perspective are endless and challenge sport scientists to uncover further patterns regarding self-esteem and physical achievement in youth sports.

## THE RELATIONSHIP BETWEEN SELF-ESTEEM
## AND PHYSICAL ACHIEVEMENT

Physical educators and sport practitioners share the enduring belief that a positive relationship exists between the development of physical skills and the enhancement of self-esteem. In essence, those who subscribe to the beneficial outcomes of sport participation agree that motor skill improvement will result in heightened levels of self-regard. Despite these claims, however, surprisingly little empirical research exists to substantiate them.

A continuing controversy among educators pertains to the causal relationship between self-esteem and achievement. Specifically, does achievement or gains in competence lead to enhanced self-esteem, or does self-esteem influence achievement? That is, does a high level of self-esteem increase the likelihood for successful accomplishment? This question of causal predominance is essential, because it suggests particular implications for curricular development in youth sport programs. Specifically, understanding the relationship between self-esteem and achievement would influence which strategies are to be used for developing these salient outcomes, competence and self-esteem, in physical activity settings.

The issue of whether self-esteem precedes achievement or vice versa elicits attention to two major theories of the self-esteem–achievement relationship. Physical educators have traditionally adopted the behaviorist or skill development view that claims gains in motor competence cause the child to emerge from the performance situation with self-views consistent with the heightened level of performance. Thus, self-esteem is basically seen as an inherent consequence of successfully mastering motor skills. The curriculum focus based on the skill development view emphasizes teaching skills and ensuring successes in competency endeavors.

Conversely, the self-consistency or self-enhancement theorists contend that self-esteem is causally predominant over achievement. Specifically, this view suggests that people tend to behave in ways and to interpret their experiences in ways that preserve or confirm self-judgments and expectations. Experiences that are compatible with the individual's evaluations of him- or herself will be accepted, and information that is inconsistent with one's self-views will be rejected. Rejection may manifest itself in such ways as discounting the success or failure or engaging in causal attributions that are compatible with one's self views. The self-consistency view has its underpinnings in the phenomenological views advanced by Combs and Snygg (1959) and Lecky (1945), who insisted upon the motivational influence of self-esteem on subsequent behavior. According to this view, curriculum recommendations focus on enhancement of self-esteem and motivation for learning in order to result in achievement gains.

A number of studies exploring the relationship between self-esteem and achievement have supported both views of causal predominance. However, an increasingly accepted view is that success experiences alone are not sufficient to enhance self-esteem if the child does not *perceive* that he or she was responsible for that success (Dweck & Elliott, 1984). Heaps (1978) expressed it well: "Real physical improvement would be useful for improving psychological well-being only to the extent information about that change is communicated and assimilated (i.e., believed)" (p. 404). The view that individuals must assume responsibility for positive outcomes in order to augment self-views is congruent with advances within the attributional framework discussed previously (Rejeski & Brawley, 1984; Weiner, 1972, 1979).

The controversy over the causal relationship between self-esteem and physical achievement nevertheless lingers on. Major reasons for this are the predominant method of employing correlational techniques to study this question and the lack of empirical studies exploring these constructs in physical settings. The remainder of this section will focus on studies that offer empirical support for both the self-consistency and skill development views.

## Self-Esteem as a Factor Influencing Achievement

Given the importance of the construct of self-esteem in both the educational and sport psychological literatures, surprisingly few studies have explored the relationship between self-esteem and achievement. Generally, investigators seeking to demonstrate the causal predominance of self-esteem over achievement have employed correlational studies (Bailey, 1971; Primavera, Simon, & Primavera, 1974; Simon & Simon, 1975). Although these and other studies report significant, positive relationships between self-esteem and academic achievement scores, and although some evidence of time precedence is apparent, the nature of such designs precludes conclusions of causal influences.

A study by Ryckman, Robbins, Thornton, and Cantrell (1982) provides some recent evidence supporting the self-enhancement model of the self-esteem–physical achievement relationship. These authors developed an instrument called the Physical Self-Efficacy Scale (PSE) to measure individuals' perceptions regarding their physical competence and expectations for success on physical tasks. To assess the predictive validity of the instrument, the investigators examined the level and extent to which a large number of students were involved in sports and the quality of their performances on a number of motor tasks. Results supported the predictive power of the PSE. Specifically, those individuals who viewed themselves as physically efficacious, in comparison to those who scored low in physical self-efficacy, participated in sports more extensively and performed at higher levels on the battery of motor tasks.

Phillips (1984) employed a rather clever design to investigate the belief that a child's perception of competence, rather than actual competence per se, is a more powerful predictor of achievement and motivated behavior. Phillips's sample consisted of 117 fifth-grade students who were all highly competent as determined by standard achievement test scores at or above the 75th national percentile. Using scores from Harter's perceived cognitive competence scale, Phillips then categorized children as accurate (high) or inaccurate (low) raters of their competence while controlling for actual ability. A number of measures were administered to the students and their teachers to provide convergent evidence regarding the children's subjective standards and expectancies; motivational orientation in terms of locus of control and achievement-related attributions; and actual classroom achievement behaviors as indicated by challenge seeking, persistence, and independent problem solving. Results offered compelling evidence for the notion that strong abilities do not guarantee feelings of personal adequacy or optimal achievement orientations. Specifically, students with low, inaccurate perceptions of their academic competence set less demanding standards of achievement and aspired to lower levels of performance; were more likely to attribute their high grades to luck and low grades to lack of ability; and were portrayed by teachers as less persistent when confronted with difficult tasks.

Four studies to date have employed causal modeling procedures to test the predictions of self-consistency theory (Felson, 1984; Shavelson & Bolus, 1981; Shewchuk & Weiss, 1986; Weiss et al., 1986). These procedures are valuable to researchers attempting to demonstrate cause-effect relationships, especially those using nonexperimental designs. A number of causal modeling approaches are available, including path analysis, cross-lagged panel correlations, simultaneous equation systems, and linear causal analysis. These techniques are especially well suited for theory testing, for allowing researchers to observe conditional events in a nonobtrusive manner, and for testing specific hypothesized causal relationships among a set of variables.

Shewchuk and Weiss (1986) devised a causal model specifying the predominance of self-esteem over achievement in a physical setting. Specifically, they hypothesized that evaluative self-perceptions of preadolescent boys and girls would exert a causal influence on their physical performance and subjective evaluations from peers. Further, anxiety was hypothesized to negatively influence physical performance and peer evaluations. The results revealed that for boys only, the causal effects of anxiety on physical performance were significant, whereas for girls, the causal influence of self-esteem on physical performance and peer evaluations was significant. For both boys and girls, however, the goodness-of-fit of the data to the causal model indicated a plausible representation of the processes responsible for causing the observed behaviors. The authors concluded that a possible reason for the lack of causal significance of self-esteem on achievement for boys may likely be that the self-esteem measure was developed primarily for use within the school environment and thus may be argued to be biased toward females.

In research mentioned previously, Weiss, Bredemeier, and Shewchuk (1986) designed a study based on the self-consistency motive as well as competence motivation theory. They formulated a causal model describing the interrelationships among perceived physical competence, perceived control, motivational orientation (challenge, criteria, curiosity), and actual competence as indicated by teachers' ratings. The results revealed that the causal data adequately fit the model and thus supported the causal precedence of self-esteem over achievement. Specifically, perceptions of one's physical competence appeared to causally influence both physical achievement and motivational orientation.

Felson (1984) recently studied the self-consistency motive in the cognitive domain both causally and longitudinally. Similar to Weiss et al., he examined the effect of self-appraisals of academic ability on academic performance (grade point average) as well as the effect of effort and anxiety as mediators of the self-appraisal–academic performance relationship. Results supported the self-consistency theory in that self-appraisals were found to have a causal, moderate effect on later academic performance, and this was partly mediated by effort.

Students who believed they were smart worked harder than students with less favorable self-appraisals, and this effort resulted in higher grades.

The implications of the findings supporting the self-consistency or self-enhancement view are clear: Actual competence is not the best predictor of future achievement and motivated behavior. One's perceptions of ability and the ensuing causal attributions appear to have a much more influential effect on achievement. This was insightfully demonstrated in the Phillips (1984) study where highly competent children who eschewed these abilities were observed to set lower standards of success, use debilitating attributions, and give up in the face of adverse conditions. Langer (1979) labels this phenomenon the "illusion of incompetence" that triggers a spiral of misperceptions and behavioral confirmations that distinguish self-doubting from confident children. Merely providing success experiences will not change these children's perceptions of incompetence. They will likely discount such experiences as attributable to luck or some other factor outside their personal control. Thus the spiral continues. Strategies are needed to create self-affirming orientations in children's views of their achievement potential.

## Achievement as a Factor Influencing Self-Esteem

Not all individuals are convinced of the strength of the self-consistency stance regarding self-esteem and achievement. The behaviorist would argue that skill development causes the child to emerge from a performance situation with self-views consistent with that particular level of performance. Physical educators and sport practitioners have been notable supporters of the skill development position, perhaps because the profession focuses primarily on the teaching of motor skills and strategies.

A number of studies using causal analysis designs have found support for the behavioristic or skill development model. Calsyn and Kenny (1977) employed 5 years of data in a cross-lagged panel model and found that the causal effect of grade point average on self-appraisals of ability is stronger than the effect of self-appraisals on grades.

Harter and Connell (1982) examined the relationships among perceived competence, perceived control, motivational orientation, and academic achievement in 784 children in Grades 3 through 9. They found that perceived control was a causal predictor of achievement, and achievement in turn causally influenced perceived competence and intrinsic motivation. Specifically, this model implies that the child who indicates an understanding of the reasons for his or her successes and failures is critical in how that child processes and reacts affectively to his or her school performance. Although the findings of this study clearly indicate support for the behavioristic view, Harter and Connell direct most of their comments to the importance of the perceived control construct as it relates to future behavior and perceived competence. Specifically, they state that when children's understanding of why they succeed and fail improves, their level of achievement and self-evaluations also improve. Children's *perceptions* of reality regarding what is responsible for their successful and unsuccessful endeavors are the most important links to future achievement and self-esteem.

Studies do exist, then, that support both the skill development and the self-consistency views. However, factors common to findings for both approaches are critical to effecting change in self-esteem and achievement behavior. First, competence gains provide the child with a salient source of information regarding his or her worth in that particular achievement domain. Second, success or skill improvements alone are not enough to change self-esteem. Rather, the child must recognize the contingencies underlying the success and accept responsibility (learn skills fast, make improvements daily, practice hard, have good skills) for success to occur. Finally, feedback and reinforcement from significant others that entail appropriate attributions for outcomes will be most valuable in shaping self-evaluations. Taken together, enhancing self-esteem requires the combination of successful mastery attempts, appropriate and adaptive attributions for success and failure, and contingent feedback by significant others.

## IMPLICATIONS FOR SPORT PRACTITIONERS

A number of recommendations for delivering sport and physical activity programs to children can be provided, based on findings reported in the previous section as well as knowledge about the development of self-esteem. Importantly, a multifactor approach to enhancing self-esteem must be adopted—one that entails the careful integration of program development, feedback and reinforcement, and the learner's self-perceptions.

### Feedback and Reinforcement

Harter's competence motivation theory and recent sport research (Horn, 1985, 1986) suggest that the quantity and quality of feedback and reinforcement from significant others influence a child's perceptions of competence. The feedback that children receive in physical settings provides a salient source of information regarding their capabilities and worth. This may be especially true for elementary-aged children who seem to depend more on social evaluation cues than do older children, as well as for children who have inaccurate and low estimations of perceived in relation to actual competence (Horn & Hasbrook, 1986; Phillips, 1984).

In light of the role of adult evaluation as a source of information for children's judgments of competence, sport practitioners should pay close attention to the absolute and relative amounts of reinforcement they give, the contingency of their reinforcement to behavior, and the attributional content of their responses to successful outcomes as well as skill errors. With regard to number and contingency of reinforcements, Horn (1986) summarizes research that has found that excessive praise given for success at an easy task or for mediocre performance is likely to convey low expectations by the evaluator to the performer. This should result in lowered perceived competence on the part of the recipient. Similarly, frequent criticism in the form of skill-corrective feedback may convey to the athlete that higher levels of achievement are expected and attainable. Despite these facts, Horn (1985) found that coaches were more likely to give high amounts of reinforcement that were noncontingent or inappropriate to low expectancy players and high amounts of criticism to high expectancy players.

## Attributions for Performance

This chapter has highlighted the importance of attributions that children use to explain their successful and unsuccessful outcomes as a means for the child to maintain and preserve his or her integrity of the self. In addition, both Harter and Connell (1982) and Weiss et al. (1986) found that perceived control, signifying the degree of understanding between one's behavior and the outcomes of that behavior, was the most potent predictor of perceived competence, actual competence, and motivated behavior. Thus, an understanding of the contingencies underlying performance outcomes is essential to psychological growth and skill-competence gains.

When coaches consider a personal, relatively stable factor such as ability as responsible for a child's success in dealing with sport skills, the child comes to expect success in future, analogous situations and acquires a positive attitude toward future participation. Assigning responsibility to external factors such as luck or task ease should not have this effect. Conversely, providing attributional feedback expressed as lack of effort or practice for skill errors implies that future attempts are not necessarily subject to the same outcome. Effort and practice are under the control of the child and can thus be changed.

Dweck and her colleagues (see Dweck & Elliott, 1984) have written extensively of attributions and their relation to achievement and motivated behavior. They have noted that children who acquire nonadaptive patterns of explaining their successes and failures come to be "learned helpless" in their approach to achievement-related endeavors. They do not see a relationship between their behavior and the eventual outcome. More importantly, Dweck and her colleagues have found that structuring success experiences alone is not sufficient to effect changes in motivated behavior, attitude, or assignment of responsibility to outcome. An effective method was to build in failures as well as successes and teach children functional ways for attributing their performances. These would be unstable, controllable factors for unsuccessful outcomes (e.g., degree of effort). This procedure is called *attribution retraining* and has far-reaching implications for educators' patterns of feedback for outcomes in children's sport.

**Instructional Strategies**

Instructional strategies most appropriate for effecting self-esteem change can be classified as *optimal challenges*, a phrase coined by Harter (1978). An optimal challenge refers to carefully matching task difficulty to the learner's developmental capabilities or, in other words, changing the activity to fit the child rather than the child to the activity. Children and adolescents derive the greatest sense of pleasure and accomplishment from having mastered skills or strategies "optimal" to their potential abilities. Succeeding at a task or skill below the optimal may likely lead to attributions of task ease and those above the optimal to luck, along with feelings of frustration. The net result is that self-esteem does not change. Designing activities to provide an optimal degree of challenge involves (a) constructing developmental sequences, (b) sequencing instructional strategies, (c) focusing on learning as opposed to performance goals, and (d) allowing for indirect teaching styles.

Constructing developmental sequences on the part of the sport practitioner entails careful analysis of the skills to be learned during the designated time period. Ordering skills from simple to complex and also making intraskill modifications to accommodate slower and faster learners can be invaluable processes for the practitioner dealing with groups of children and adolescents. Inter- and intraskill sequences and strategies allow for the mastering of skills at each individual's level and rate of learning. Instructors can structure practice situations more easily to accommodate the variety of developmental levels found in each classroom.

Sequencing instructional strategies, a method for optimizing skill acquisition and self-esteem, emerges from literature on developmental levels of motor control (Bressan & Woollacott, 1982). Developmental sequencing consists of four phases:

1. Children explore qualities of moving (see Logsdon et al., 1984).

2. Demonstrations and practice of single skills or skill combinations are provided.

3. Children design activity sequences or games according to certain parameters.

4. Demonstrations and practice of more complex skills and strategies are provided.

The third developmental phase in this sequence, formally called the *accommodating level*, explicitly tackles the issue of enhancing self-esteem. At this level, children are given opportunities to design their own routines and activities given certain parameters, both individually and in groups. They are also allowed to make decisions on when and how to use the skills in their routine or sequence. This strategy is self-enhancing by giving children *control* over their environment and by providing concrete evidence for helping the child understand the contingencies between his or her actions and resultant change in behavior. When children are involved in designing their own activities, optimal challenges are likely. Thus, successful mastery should be attributed to ability or skill improvement and unsuccessful attempts to lack of practice.

A number of researchers in both the educational (see Dweck & Elliott, 1984) and sport psychological (Burton, 1983; Gould, 1986) disciplines have noted the importance of learning or process goals versus outcome or product goals as they affect achievement and psychosocial growth. The primary focus of learning goals is to increase competence or to improve relative to one's own past performance. Outcome goals focus on the results of one's performance (e.g., grade on a test, score of a contest, win-loss). In addition, Dweck and Elliott (1984) note that children who are primarily oriented toward outcome goals are interested in obtaining favorable judgment of competence or avoiding a negative judgment of competence by significant others. Seeking to learn versus seeking to obtain competence judgments, they say, leads children to process information about their performance differently. Children with a learning-goal orientation ask the questions, How can I do it? and What will I learn?; whereas those with an outcome orientation focus on Can I do it? (e.g., win) and Will I look good (smart)?

Burton (1983) suggests that the critical aspect of process goals is that they are flexible and under the athlete's control. Children and adolescents can participate in setting their goals in a number of skill areas according to realistic expectations of improvement and performance. As athletes master their goals, responsibility should be assigned to the self in terms of ability, whereas unsuccessful mastery can result in adjusting the process goal in order to provide an optimal challenge. Thus, when properly employed, process goals result in enhanced levels of self-esteem, motivation, and ultimately performance.

Closely aligned with sequencing instructional strategies and goal orientation are interactional styles of instruction. Instructional styles can range on a continuum from direct and controlling to indirect and autonomous (Mosston, 1981). Recently, a great deal has been written with regard to the positive effects of more indirect and autonomous teaching styles in order to enhance self-esteem, intrinsic motivation, and achievement (Deci, Sheinman, Schwartz, & Ryan, 1981; Dweck & Elliott, 1984; Harter, 1981c; Logsdon et al., 1984). With this approach, children are allowed to use problem-solving methods of inquiry about skill mastery and to engage in decision making regarding when and how to use skills and strategies. As mentioned before, this style of instruction lets children control their environment and provides them with more realistic expectations of performance. In addition, Dweck and Elliott (1984) have found that instructors who favor a process or learning-goal orientation for the child are likely to act more as resources rather than judges, to focus children more on process than outcome, to react to errors as natural and useful rather than as failures, to stress effort and personal standards rather than ability and normative standards, and to stimulate achievement through intrinsic as opposed to extrinsic strategies.

Deci et al. (1981) have demonstrated the strength of this stance. These researchers first devised an instrument to assess teachers' orientations toward control versus autonomy with children. They found that students in Grades 4 through 6 reliably rated their teachers as controlling or autonomous as the scale indicated. Students of autonomy-oriented teachers were more intrinsically motivated (i.e., process-oriented) and had higher self-esteem at the end of the year than did students of teachers with control orientations. These findings pertaining to self-esteem development suggest that practitioners of children's sport and physical activity consider alternative styles of teaching other than the traditional direct and controlling style found in organized youth sports.

## Developing Observation Skills

A final recommendation with regard to enhancing self-esteem and subsequent physical achievement is that teachers and coaches develop their own observation skills in physical settings. Barrett (1983) has noted that the ability to observe behaviors and performance in a physical setting is critical in order for instructors to give appropriate, contingent, skill-relevant feedback. Unfortunately, practitioners often take observation skills for granted. However, knowing that children low in self-esteem behave differently in learning situations and are more sensitive to certain sources of information than others, instructors must be aware of children who manifest differing levels of perceived competence in their classrooms. Behaviors descriptive of the low self-esteem child include avoiding activities, giving up easily when trying to learn new skills, exerting minimal effort in games and activities, setting unrealistic performance standards (too low or too high), attributing success to luck and failure to lack of ability, and adopting strategies to avoid failure (making excuses, not feeling good, etc.). When instructors become attuned to these overt behaviors, they in turn can respond with the appropriate strategies to enhance self-esteem and motivation discussed earlier.

## CONCLUDING REMARKS

Self-esteem emerges out of social interactions and thus merits the attention of sport scientists and practitioners. Self-esteem development must become part of the explicit, not hidden, agenda of our instructional practices, by leading us to focus on strategies targeted to enhance self-esteem and consequently motivation and achievement. These strategies include using appropriate feedback and reinforcement, helping children understand the contingencies underlying their behavior and subsequent performance, focusing on optimal challenges, including developmental sequences, sequencing instructional strategies and indirect teaching styles, and focusing on a process-goal orientation rather than an outcome orientation. Thus, building in success experiences is not sufficient for positively influencing self-esteem. Children must perceive and believe that their actions are responsible for the success and that they can control skill improvement and successful outcomes. Teachers, coaches, and parents can only accomplish this by understanding the strategies that are conducive to effecting change in self-esteem, with the ultimate outcomes being improved motivation and physical achievement.

## *Acknowledgments*

I want to express my deepest appreciation to my students and colleagues who generously gave their time to review an earlier version of this manuscript. Heartfelt thanks go to Bob Brustad, Kim Klint, Elizabeth Bressan, Daniel Gould, and Mary Faeth Chenery. A special thank you goes to Don Morris for keeping me on my toes in terms of the ''real world'' of elementary physical education, and to Thelma Horn for providing critical amounts of contingent and appropriate feedback at various phases during the writing of this chapter.

## REFERENCES

Bailey, R.C. (1971). Self-concept differences in low and high achieving students. *Journal of Clinical Psychology, 27*, 188–190.

Bandura, A. (1977). Self-efficacy: Toward a unifying theory for behavioral change. *Psychological Review, 84*, 191–215.

Barrett, K.R. (1983). A hypothetical model of observing as a teaching skill. *Journal of Teaching in Physical Education, 3*, 22–31.

Bressan, E.S., & Woollacott, M.H. (1982). A prescriptive paradigm for sequencing instruction in physical education. *Human Movement Science, 1*, 155–175.

Burton, D. (1983). *Evaluation of goal setting training on selected cognitions and performance of collegiate swimmers*. Unpublished doctoral dissertation, University of Illinois, Urbana.

Calsyn, R.J., & Kenny, D.A. (1977). Self-concept of ability and perceived evaluation of others: Cause or effect of academic achievement? *Journal of Educational Psychology, 69*, 136–145.

Coakley, J.J. (1984, July). *Mead's theory on the development of the self: Implications for organized youth sport programs*. Paper presented at the Olympic Scientific Congress, Eugene, OR.

Coleman, J.S. (1961). *The adolescent society: The social life of the teenager and its impact on education*. New York: Free Press.

Combs, A.W., & Snygg, D. (1959). *Individual behavior: A perceptual approach to behavior*. New York: Harper.

Connell, J.P. (1980). *A multidimensional measure of children's perceptions of control*. Denver: University of Denver.

Connell, J.P. (1985). A new multidimensional measure of children's perceptions of control. *Child Development,* **56**(4), 1018–1041.

Cooley, C.H. (1902/1956). *Human nature and the social order*. Glencoe, IL: Free Press.

Coopersmith, S. (1967). *The antecedents of self-esteem*. San Francisco: W.H. Freeman.

Covington, L.V., & Beery, R.G. (1977). *Self-worth and school learning*. New York: Holt, Rinehart, & Winston.

Deci, E.L., Sheinman, L., Schwartz, A.J., & Ryan, R.M. (1981). An instrument to assess adult's orientations toward control versus autonomy with children: Reflections on intrinsic motivation and perceived competence. *Journal of Educational Psychology,* **23**, 642–650.

Diener, C.J., & Dweck, C.S. (1978). An analysis of learned helplessness: Continuous changes in performance strategy, and achievement cognitions following failure. *Journal of Personality and Social Psychology,* **36**, 451–462.

Dweck, C.S., & Elliott, E.S. (1984). Achievement motivation. In M. Hetherington (Ed.), *Social development: Carmichael's manual in child psychology* (pp. 643–691). New York: Wiley.

Eitzen, D.S. (1976). Athletes in the status system of male adolescents: A replication of Coleman's *The Adolescent Society*. In A. Yiannakis, T.D. McIntyre, M.J. Melnick, & D.P. Hart (Eds.), *Sport sociology: Contemporary themes* (2nd ed., pp. 150–154). Dubuque, IA: Kendall-Hunt.

Epstein, S. (1973). The self-concept revisited or a theory of a theory. *American Psychologist,* **28**, 404–416.

Felson, R.B. (1984). The effect of self-appraisals of ability on academic performance. *Journal of Personality and Social Psychology,* **47**, 944–952.

Feltz, D.L. (1978). Athletics in the status system of female adolescents. *Review of Sport and Leisure*, 98–108.

Feltz, D.L., & Petlichkoff, L. (1983). Perceived competence among interscholastic sport participants and dropouts. *Canadian Journal of Applied Sport Sciences,* **8**, 231–235.

Gecas, V. (1982). The self-concept. *Annual Review of Sociology,* **8**, 1–33.

Gould, D. (1986). Goal setting for peak performance. In J. Williams (Ed.), *Sport psychology for coaches: Personal growth to peak performance* (pp. 133–148). Palo Alto, CA: Mayfield.

Gould, D., Horn, T., & Spreeman, J. (1983). Competitive anxiety in junior elite wrestlers. *Journal of Sport Psychology,* **5**, 58–71.

Harter, S. (1974). Pleasure derived from cognitive challenge and mastery. *Child Development,* **45**, 661–669.

Harter, S. (1978). Effectance motivation reconsidered. *Human Development,* **21**, 34–64.

Harter, S. (1981a). The development of competence motivation in the mastery of cognitive and physical skills: Is there still a place for joy? In C.H. Nadeau (Ed.), *Psychology of motor behavior and sport—1980* (pp. 3–29). Champaign, IL: Human Kinetics.

Harter, S. (1981b). A model of intrinsic mastery motivation in children: Individual differences and developmental change. In W.A. Collins (Ed.), *Minnesota Symposium on Child Psychology* (Vol. 14, pp. 215–255). Hillsdale, NJ: Erlbaum.

Harter, S. (1981c). A new self-report scale of intrinsic versus extrinsic orientation in the classroom: Motivational and informational components. *Developmental Psychology,* **17**(3), 300–312.

Harter, S. (1982a). A developmental perspective on some parameters of self-regulation in children. In P. Karoly & F.H. Karger (Eds.), *Self-management and behavioral change: From theory to practice.* Elmsford, NY: Pergamon Press.

Harter, S. (1982b). The perceived competence scale for children. *Child Development,* **53**, 87–97.

Harter, S. (1983). The development of the self-system. In M. Hetherington (Ed.), *Handbook of child psychology: Social and personality development* (Vol. 4). New York: Wiley.

Harter, S. (1985). Competence as a dimension of self-evaluation: Toward a comprehensive model of self-worth. In R. Leahy (Ed.), *The development of the self* (pp. 55–121). New York: Academic Press.

Harter, S., & Connell, J.P. (1982). A comparison of alternative models of the relationship between academic achievement and children's perceptions of competence, control, and motivational orientation. In J. Nicholls (Ed.), *The development of achievement-related cognitions and behaviors* (pp. 153–197). Greenwich, CT: JAI Press.

Harter, S., & Pike, R. (1983). *The pictorial scale of perceived competence and social acceptance for young children.* Denver: University of Denver.

Heaps, R.A. (1978). Relating physical and psychological fitness: A psychological point of view. *Journal of Sports Medicine and Physical Fitness,* **18**, 399–408.

Horn, T.S. (1985). Coaches' feedback and changes in children's perceptions of their physical competence. *Journal of Educational Psychology, 77*, 174–186.

Horn, T.S. (1986). The self-fulfilling prophecy theory: When coaches' expectations become reality. In J. Williams (Ed.), *Sport psychology for coaches: Personal growth to peak performance* (pp. 59–73). Palo Alto, CA: Mayfield.

Horn, T.S., & Hasbrook, C.A. (1986). Informational components influencing children's perceptions of their physical competence. In M.R. Weiss & D. Gould (Eds.), *Sport for children and youths* (pp. 81–88). Champaign, IL: Human Kinetics.

Horn, T.S., & Weiss, M.R. (1986, June). *A developmental analysis of children's self-ability judgements*. Paper presented at the annual meeting of the North American Society for the Psychology of Sport and Physical Activity, Scottsdale, AZ.

James, W. (1890). *The principles of psychology*. New York: Henry Holt.

Kirchner, G. (1985). *Physical education for elementary school children* (6th ed.). Dubuque, IA: Wm. C. Brown.

Klint, K.A. (1985). *Participation motives and self-perceptions of current and former athletes in youth gymnastics*. Unpublished master's thesis, University of Oregon, Eugene.

Klint, K.A., & Weiss, M.R. (in press). *Perceived competence and motives for participating in youth gymnastics: A test of Harter's competence motivation theory*. Manuscript submitted for publication.

Langer, E.J. (1979). The illusion of incompetence. In L.C. Perlmutter & R.A. Monty (Eds.), *Choice and perceived control*. Hillsdale, NJ: Erlbaum.

Lecky, P. (1945). *Self-consistency: A theory of personality*. Long Island, NY: Island Press.

Logsdon, B.J., Barrett, K.R., Ammons, M., Broer, M.R., Halvorson, L.E., McGee, R., & Roberton, M.A. (1984). *Physical education for children: A focus on the teaching process*. Philadelphia: Lea & Febiger.

Martens, R., Christina, R.W., Sharkey, B.S., & Harvey, J.S. (1981). *Coaching young athletes*. Champaign, IL: Human Kinetics.

Mead, G.H. (1934). *Mind, self, and society*. Chicago: University of Chicago Press.

Minton, B. (1979, April). *Dimensions of information underlying children's judgments of their competence*. Paper presented at the meeting of Society for Research for Child Development, San Francisco, CA.

Morris, G.S.D., & Stiehl, J. (1985). *Physical education: From intent to action*. Columbus, OH: Merrill.

Mosston, M. (1981). *Teaching physical education* (2nd ed.). Columbus, OH: Merrill.

Nowicki, S., & Strickland, B. (1973). A locus of control scale for children. *Journal of Consulting and Clinical Psychology, 40*, 148–154.

Passer, M.W. (1984). Competence trait anxiety in children and adolescents. In J.M. Silva & R.S. Weinberg (Eds.), *Psychological foundations of sport* (pp. 130–144). Champaign, IL: Human Kinetics.

Phillips, D. (1984). The illusion of incompetence among academically competent children. *Child Development, 55*, 2000–2016.

Primavera, L.H., Simon, W.E., & Primavera, A.M. (1974). The relationship between self-esteem and academic achievement: An investigation of sex differences. *Psychology in the Schools, 11*, 213–216.

Rejeski, W.J., & Brawley, L.R. (1984). Attribution theory in sport. *Journal of Sport Psychology, 5*, 77–99.

Roberts, G.C., Kleiber, D.A., & Duda, J.L. (1981). An analysis of motivation in children's sport: The role of perceived competence in participation. *Journal of Sport Psychology, 3*, 206–216.

Rosenberg, M. (1979). *Conceiving the self.* New York: Basic Books.

Ruble, D.N., Boggiano, A.K., Feldman, N.S., & Loebl, J.H. (1980). Developmental analysis of the role of social comparison in self-evaluation. *Developmental Psychology, 16*, 105–115.

Ryckman, R.M., Robbins, M.A., Thornton, B., & Cantrell, P. (1982). Development and validation of a physical self-efficacy scale. *Journal of Personality and Social Psychology, 42*, 891–900.

Scanlan, T.K. (1982). Social evaluation: A key developmental element in the competition process. In R.A. Magill, M.J. Ash, & F.L. Smoll (Eds.), *Children in sport: A contemporary anthology* (pp. 138–152). Champaign, IL: Human Kinetics.

Scanlan, T.K., & Lewthwaite, R. (1984). Social psychological aspects of competition for male youth sport participants: I. Predictors of competitive stress. *Journal of Sport Psychology, 6*, 208–226.

Scanlan, T.K., & Lewthwaite, R. (1986). Social psychological aspects of competition for male youth sport participants: IV. Predictors of enjoyment. *Journal of Sport Psychology, 8*, 25–35.

Scanlan, T.K., & Passer, M.W. (1978). Factors related to competitive stress among male youth sport participants. *Medicine and Science in Sports, 109*, 103–108.

Scanlan, T.K., & Passer, M.W. (1979). Sources of competitive stress in young female athletes. *Journal of Sport Psychology, 1*, 151–159.

Shavelson, R.J., & Bolus, R. (1981). *Self-concept: The interplay of theory and methods*. Santa Monica, CA: Rand.

Shavelson, R.J., Hubner, J.J., & Stanton, G.C. (1976). Self-concept validation of construct interpretations. *Review of Educational Research, 46*, 407–441.

Shewchuk, R.M., & Weiss, M.R. (1986). *Self-concept and physical performance of preadolescent children: A causal analysis*. Unpublished manuscript, University of Oregon, Eugene.

Simon, W.E., & Simon, M.G. (1975). Self-esteem, intelligence and standardized academic achievement. *Psychology in the Schools, 12*, 97–100.

Ulrich, B.D. (in press). Perceptions of physical competence and motor competence as correlates to motivation to participate in sport in young children. *Research Quarterly for Exercise and Sport*.

Vallerand, R.J. (1983). On emotion in sport: Theoretical and social psychological perspectives. *Journal of Sport Psychology, 5*, 197–215.

Wankel, L.M., & Kreisel, P.S.J. (1985). Factors underlying enjoyment of youth sports: Sport and age group comparisons. *Journal of Sport and Psychology, 7*, 51–64.

Weiner, B. (1972). Attribution theory, achievement motivation and the educational process. *Review of Educational Research, 42*(2), 203–215.

Weiner, B. (1979). A theory of motivation for some classroom experiences. *Journal of Educational Psychology, 71*, 3–25.

Weiss, M.R., & Bredemeier, B.J. (1983). Developmental sport psychology: A theoretical perspective for studying children in sport. *Journal of Sport Psychology, 5*, 216–230.

Weiss, M.R., Bredemeier, B.J., & Shewchuk, R.M. (1985). An intrinsic/extrinsic motivation scale for the youth sport setting: A confirmatory factor analysis. *Journal of Sport Psychology, 7*, 75–91.

Weiss, M.R., Bredemeier, B.J., & Shewchuk, R.M. (1986). The dynamics of perceived competence, perceived control, and motivational orientation in youth sports. In M.R. Weiss & D. Gould (Eds.), *Sport for children and youths* (pp. 89–101). Champaign, IL: Human Kinetics.

Weiss, M.R., & Shewchuk, R.M. (1985, May). *The motivational orientation in sport scale: A replication and validation*. Paper presented at the annual meeting of the North American Society for the Psychology of Sport and Physical Activity, Gulf Park, MS.

Wells, L.E., & Marwell, G. (1976). *Self-esteem: Its conceptualization and measurement*. Beverly Hills, CA: Sage.

White, R. (1959). Motivation reconsidered: The concept of competence. *Psychological Review, 66*, 297–333.

Williams, J.M., & White, K.A. (1985). Adolescent status systems for males and females at three age levels. *Adolescence.*

Wylie, R.C. (1979). *The self-concept: Theory and research on selected topics* (Vol. 2). Lincoln: University of Nebraska Press.

# 6

# The Influence
# of Teacher-Coach Behavior
# on the Psychological
# Development of Children

Thelma Sternberg Horn

Within the last decade, several theories have appeared in the developmental and educational psychology literature that attempt to explain the processes by which children develop certain achievement-oriented psychological characteristics (e.g., Cooper & Good, 1983; Harter, 1981; McCombs, 1984; Schunk, 1984; Wang, 1983). These characteristics include intrinsic motivation, high self-concept, an internal locus of control, and low performance anxiety. Each of the theorists listed above, in formulating his or her respective conceptual model, has specifically identified the behavior of significant adults as one of the primary factors influencing the degree to which children will acquire such positive characteristics during their preadolescent years. Correspondingly, research reported within the last decade in the educational and sport science literature has provided strong *empirical* support for the hypothesized relationship between adult behavior and children's psychosocial growth in instructional settings (e.g., Horn, 1985a; Peterson, 1977; Smith, Smoll, & Curtis, 1979; Smith, Zane, Smoll, & Coppel, 1983; Smoll, Smith, Curtis, & Hunt, 1978; Solomon & Kendall, 1976). These research projects, which have generally been conducted in academic classrooms or athletic field settings, provide evidence that the behavior of the individual teacher or coach affects the psychosocial development of children above and beyond that exerted by the school, curriculum, or athletic program itself. As Coakley (1987) has concluded, there appears to be little evidence that mere participation in a youth sport program has any significant socialization effects on the child. However, sufficient research does exist to indicate that the behaviors exhibited by individual coaches within a program can affect the attitudes, values, and self-perceptions of young athletes.

This chapter presents the information from both the theoretical psychology literature and the empirically based instructional effectiveness literature to delineate the role that the teacher and coach can play in facilitating children's psychological growth through physical activity. To begin, some of the relevant psychological and educational theories that provide explanations as to *how* adults' behavior affects children's psychological responses will be examined. Then the research on instructional effectiveness will be reviewed to identify the particular adult behaviors that may be most effective or ineffective in facilitating such psychological growth.

## THEORETICAL PERSPECTIVES

The theories or conceptual models referred to in the previous section each propose that the behavior of significant adults in achievement contexts has an effect on the corresponding behavior and psychological responses of children. Susan Harter and several of her colleagues at the University of Denver, for example, have formulated a model (Harter, 1981) to explain the observed differences between children in their intrinsic motivation to pursue mastery or to become competent in the various achievement domains and identify adult feedback as an important component. Harter theorizes that the evaluative feedback given by significant adults in response to children's performance affects children's perceptions of how competent they are in that particular achievement activity. Children who receive consistent and positive adult evaluation of their performance will develop a high regard for their personal competence and their ability to control subsequent performance. High perceived competence and performance control in turn cause children to develop and exhibit such other positive attributes and behaviors as intrinsic motivation, high self-esteem, low performance anxiety, and persistence at achieving task mastery.

The notion that adult feedback serves as a source of competence information for children is a theme that is repeated in several other recently published theories concerning children's psychosocial growth in educational contexts. Dale Schunk (1984), for example, utilizes Bandura's (1977) theory of self-efficacy to explain what he has termed differential levels of *motivated learning* (i.e., motivation to acquire academic skills and knowledge) in the classroom. Consistent with Bandura's identification of persuasory feedback as one of the four sources of self-efficacy information, Schunk also identifies adult behavior as one important factor in children's development of academic self-efficacy. He postulates that certain teaching behaviors, such as the instructors' presentation of academic tasks and the quality or content of the teachers' feedback, can affect students' self-efficacy by supplying them with either positive or negative information concerning their competencies. Students' perceptions of their performance competencies in turn affect their motivation to engage in mastery behaviors.

Similarly, the various expectancy models (e.g., Brophy & Good, 1974; Cooper & Good, 1983) that were developed and extensively tested during the last decade have provided information concerning the link between teachers' behavior and children's psychological growth. The sequential steps typically outlined in these models suggest that teachers' expectations or judgments concerning the academic ability of individual students in their classroom affect the teachers' behavior towards these students. Such differential or expectancy-biased treatment of students within a class not only affects each child's opportunity to learn but also conveys differential information to the child concerning his or her competence, thus affecting the child's subsequent performance and behavior. These expectancy models hypothesize, then, that the teacher's original or initial judgment of a student's capabilities can serve as a self-fulfilling prophecy by setting in motion a series of events that ultimately cause the teacher's original expectation for each child to be fulfilled.

In addition to the models just described, several other theories regarding children's psychological development have appeared recently (e.g., McCombs, 1984; Wang, 1983). Although each of these models was actually formulated to address different aspects of children's psychological development (e.g., self-efficacy, perceived competence, intrinsic mastery behavior, perceived personal control, etc.), each contains a common theme with regard to facilitating positive psychological growth in children. This theme suggests that the verbal and non-verbal responses given by significant adults in response to a child's achievement performance provide that child with information concerning his or her competence and worth. Such evaluative information then affects the child's self-confidence, achievement motivation, level of performance anxiety, and ultimately his or her achievement performance.

These models explain *how* adult behavior affects children. However, to determine detailed and prescriptive information regarding the teacher's or coach's role, we also need to identify the *particular* adult behaviors that will be most effective in promoting positive self-perceptions in children. For example, how should the teacher respond to the winners and losers in her third-grade class after an all-school track meet? What should the coach say to a batter who has struck out for the third time in an important game? What are the effective and ineffective responses a parent can make to a child's performance attempts? To answer such questions, we need to turn to a different literature source— that containing the empirically based research on instructional effectiveness.

## RESEARCH ON INSTRUCTIONAL EFFECTIVENESS

Investigators in this area of study have for many decades attempted to identify the correlates of effective teaching. An historical examination of this rich body of research shows considerable variation across different research "eras" in the paradigms used to study teaching effectiveness. According to a review written by Medley (1979), this variation in research methodology and design is primarily due to changes that have occurred over the decades in the definition or conceptualization of what effective teaching actually is. Medley has identified three broad but distinct conceptual definitions of teaching effectiveness, each of which has been associated with a different research paradigm.

The earliest of these research orientations was based on the belief that the effectiveness of a teacher in promoting student growth was a function of the *personality traits* of the individual teacher. Therefore, research in this era was designed to identify those traits that characterized the "good" teacher and that distinguished him or her from the "poor" teacher. Although a certain amount of this type of research was conducted in the early years, results were seldom consistent across studies.

The second era in the literature on instructional effectiveness was characterized by the belief that teaching effectiveness was basically a function of the particular *teaching method or style* used in the classroom. Teaching effectiveness was investigated by comparing the effects that selected teaching techniques (e.g., "open" versus "structured") or teaching styles (e.g., "teacher-dominant" versus "guided discovery") exerted on students' academic and psychosocial growth. Although this investigative paradigm has been rather extensively used, it has not, in general, resulted in a consistent body of knowledge that can be replicated across classrooms. This lack of validity and generalizability has been attributed to the fact that the teachers' behavior within each instructional method or style is often not considered or controlled.

This criticism led to the third approach to the study of teaching effectiveness. Under this conceptual definition, teaching effectiveness is believed to be a function of the *behaviors* a teacher exhibits in instructional contexts. The research paradigm for identifying effective teaching behaviors is the process-product methodology. This paradigm requires (a) valid and reliable assessments of instructor and student behaviors in an academic context (i.e., measurement of process variables) and (b) comparable assessment of the educational product (i.e., gains in students' performance or psychological growth over the instructional unit). Initially, this research is correlational in nature as process variables (measures of teacher and student behavior) are correlated with product variables (student gain scores) to identify the effective and ineffective instructional behaviors. Ultimately, causal relationships between the process-product measures are established through sophisticated statistical techniques and/or through experimental manipulation of process variables in field or laboratory studies.

The use of this process-product paradigm in numerous research projects conducted throughout the last decade in academic and, to a lesser extent, motor skill instructional settings has resulted in rather consistent and impressive information concerning instructional behavior. In addition, researchers have used the process-product paradigm in the psychological literature to study parent-child or teacher-child relationships. Therefore, in the rest of this chapter we will use the information obtained from *both* the educational and the psychological literatures to identify and discuss possible correlates of effective instructional behavior.

## EFFECTIVE AND INEFFECTIVE INSTRUCTIONAL BEHAVIORS

The process-product methodology has been successfully employed in a variety of contexts to examine the relationship between adult behavior and children's psychological responses. Some of these investigations were field-based and primarily correlational in nature, whereas others were conducted in highly controlled laboratory contexts and were designed to test particular theoretical constructs. A careful review and synthesis of this disparate research suggest that three characteristics or components of adult behavior seem to be most consistently associated with children's psychological growth. These three behavioral components include (a) the contingency and quality of praise and criticism exhibited by adults in response to children's performance successes and failures, (b) the frequency and quality of performance-relevant information provided to children during their performance attempts, and (c) the direct or implicit attribution contained in the evaluative feedback given by adult observers.

### Contingency and Quality of Praise and Criticism

In this section, *praise* and *criticism* refer to particular types of evaluative feedback given in response to a child's performance and express the adult's approval of or disappointment in the child's performance or behavior. Expressions of praise or criticism, then, go beyond simple provision of performance feedback because they also contain the adult's affective evaluation of the worth or merit of the child's performance. Thus, in an achievement setting, praise and criticism can actually be considered to be rewards or punishment that may operate like other rewards/reinforcers (e.g., candy, money, toys, trophies, awards, etc.).

In recent years, the value of using such rewards in achievement settings has been questioned due to the field and laboratory research showing that extrinsic rewards can, under certain circumstances, actually undermine or decrease children's task motivation. According to Deci's cognitive-evaluation theory (Deci & Ryan, 1985), extrinsic rewards should facilitate children's intrinsic motivation if the administration of such awards provides them with positive information concerning their competence and if children do not perceive the reward to be controlling their behavior. Although much of the research conducted to test this theory has examined the impact of material awards on intrinsic motivation, some investigators have examined Deci's theory in laboratory settings using verbal feedback as the extrinsic reward (e.g., Anderson, Manoogian, & Reznick, 1976; Boggiano & Ruble, 1979; Pittman, Davey, Alafat, Wetherill, & Kramer, 1980; Ryan, 1982; Vallerand & Reid, 1984). The combined results of these studies indicate support for the cognitive-evaluation theory. Adult praise can serve to facilitate children's motivation but only if such feedback is administered in a noncontrolling, performance-contingent, and specific manner, thus providing the child with positive information concerning his or her competence.

Unfortunately, observational classroom research suggests that the praise teachers exhibit in a normal classroom setting is often neither specific nor given contingent on children's performance or behavior. In a general review of the research and an ensuing discussion of the function of teacher praise, Brophy (1981) concludes that many teachers do not use praise as a specific and performance-contingent reward for meritorious performance but instead may employ generalized praise as a controlling, disciplinary, or motivational tool. Not surprisingly, measures of adult praise in instructional settings have been found to be only modestly correlated, and in some cases even negatively correlated, with gains in student achievement and psychological growth (Brophy & Evertson, 1976; Good, Ebmeier, & Beckerman, 1978; Horn, 1985a; Martin, Veldman, & Anderson, 1980; Parsons, Kaczala, & Meece, 1982).

Furthermore, analysis of the distribution of such noncontingent praise within each class has shown that certain children may receive more generalized and noncontingent praise than do their classmates. The observational classroom data collected by several researchers (e.g., Brookover, Schweitzer, Schneider, Beady, Flood, & Wisenbaker, 1978; Kleinfeld, 1975; Weinstein, 1976) showed that children who the teacher perceived to be low-ability students received proportionately more inappropriate praise than children who were perceived to be of higher ability. These results suggest that some teachers may be trying to balance the amount of praise they give individual children in the classroom by providing all students with an equal amount of praise, even when their performance is not equally meritorious. Unfortunately, this well-intentioned instructional strategy may not be effective as it may often mean that the lower ability students are receiving inappropriate and noncontingent feedback.

**Feedback contingency and children's self-perceptions.** According to Deci's theory (Deci & Ryan, 1985), noncontingent praise might undermine children's motivation because it is perceived to be controlling and provides children with no information concerning their competence. However, recent research reported in the educational literature suggests that noncontingent or inappropriate praise, as administered by adults to certain children in a *group* setting, can actually convey *negative* information concerning these children's competence. These results were consistently found in a series of studies conducted by Meyer and his colleagues (Meyer et al., 1979; Meyer, Mittag, & Engler, 1985). In the earlier studies in this series, subjects from various age groups were given written vignettes that depicted two performers who had achieved the same level of performance (either successful or unsuccessful outcomes) but who received differential feedback from an adult evaluator. In the success condition, one of the individuals was described as having received neutral feedback from the adult (e.g., "That's correct"), whereas the other performer received more extensive praise for the same performance. Despite the fact that both performers were equally successful, subjects perceived the performer who received neutral praise to be higher in ability than the second one who received more extensive praise. In the failure condition, one performer received criticism as the adult response to the unsuccessful performance, whereas the other received neutral feedback (e.g., "That's incorrect"). Again, based only on such differential feedback, subjects believed the performer who received critical feedback to be the individual with the greater ability. Meyer et al. (1979) explained these results by suggesting that the differential feedback conveyed information regarding the adult's evaluation of the two students' competence. The comparably greater praise given one performer for an easy success suggested that the adult thought that performer to have lesser ability and thus had established a lower performance standard. Similarly, criticism or blame given for an individual's failure, in contrast to the neutral feedback given to a coperformer, implied that the adult believed the criticized individual to have higher ability and thus to be capable of improved performance.

In two subsequent studies (Meyer et al., 1985), these researchers continued their examination of this phenomenon by employing a laboratory protocol in which two "students" (subjects) were administered an academic task by two "teachers" (confederates of the experimenter). These teacher-confederates provided differential feedback to the student-subjects who had actually attained identical levels of successful or unsuccessful performance. Under conditions in which the "teachers" were presumed to have prior knowledge about the subject's capabilities (i.e., simulating a typical classroom situation), the student-subjects who received comparably greater praise for successes and neutral feedback (no blame) for failures perceived themselves to have lower ability than their coperformer who had obtained identical performance scores but had received neutral feedback (no praise) for successes and criticism (blame) for failures.

In discussing the combined results of this series of studies, Meyer et al. (1985) suggested that the effects of adult praise and blame in instructional settings may not be as straightforward as reinforcement theory suggests (i.e., that praise should facilitate and criticism should decrease student motivation). Rather the impact of this type of feedback from teachers may be mediated by the contingency of the praise or criticism (i.e., the level of performance for which it is given) and by the students' cognitive interpretation of that feedback. In a group setting, the teacher's or coach's use of praise and criticism will be interpreted by each performer relative to the evaluative feedback received by comparison others.

The impact of differential adult feedback may be particularly relevant in motor skill instructional settings where the quality of a child's performance can easily be distinguished from that of comparison others. If a teacher or coach responds to a particular child's performance with effusive praise even when the child and his or her class or teammates clearly believe that the performance was no better than that of comparison others, then information is conveyed to the child that he or she has less competence than those peers. Thus, the patterns of reinforcement exhibited by the teacher or coach may be establishing a certain level of performance expectations for each child. Effusive praise given to a particular child for a mediocre level of performance (e.g., getting a walk on four wild pitches) or for success at an easy task (e.g., catching an easy infield pop-up) implies that that is the maximum level of performance expected of that athlete. In contrast, his or her class or teammate who is given less effusive or no praise for an easy or mediocre performance is indirectly being told that he or she is capable of reaching a higher level of performance. Similarly, providing a performer with criticism after a performance error may convey high competence information. However, the child whose skill errors are consistently ignored by the teacher or coach may believe that he or she is incapable of improving (i.e., has low competence).

These comments regarding both the impact of differential instructional feedback and the relative "value" of criticism as an effective adult response to a child's performance errors are offered with some caution at this point for two reasons. First, as Meyer et al. (1979) have demonstrated, the negative impact of differential adult feedback does not generalize to young children who are perhaps cognitively incapable of inferring differential levels of personal ability from differential adult feedback for the same level of performance. The research of Meyer and his colleagues (1979) showed that a majority of their sample of children in Grades 3 to 5 judged the "student" who received praise from the teacher after successes and no criticism after failures to be higher in ability than the "student" who received neutral praise and more extensive blame. Younger children, particularly those under age 10, may be more apt to interpret adult praise and criticism in a literal or straightforward manner, whereas older children do not. Such developmental differences in regard to the effectiveness of certain instructional behaviors will be discussed more fully later in this chapter.

Second, caution should also be advocated with regard to the "value" of criticism as an effective response to a child's performance errors. Although some criticism may connote a higher performance expectation for the child and thus promote positive perceptions of competence, very high frequencies of criticism may establish a standard of performance that is too high and that the child feels incapable of reaching. This pattern of evaluative feedback from parents (i.e., high frequencies of negative reinforcement and few expressions of performance-contingent praise) has been implicated in the social psychology literature (e.g., Dusek, 1980; Krohne, 1980) as one factor that may contribute to the development of high trait anxiety during the childhood years. In the sport research as well, high competitive trait anxious children have been found to expect failure-contingent negative evaluation from significant adults more than do their low competitive trait anxious peers (Passer, 1983). Thus, an optimal level or ratio of praise and criticism may exist that will be most effective for children, with extremes in either direction (e.g., high praise and minimal criticism or minimal praise and high criticism) being detrimental.

**Feedback contingency and children's performance evaluations.** As a final point in regard to the impact of evaluative feedback, it should also be noted that adults' praise and criticism in achievement settings may affect children's perceptions regarding *how* their performance is to be evaluated. Ames and Ames (1984), citing their research investigating the effects of a competitive goal-structure versus a cooperative or individualistic goal-orientation on children's self-perceptions, point out that children working under competitive reward conditions are more apt to depend on social comparison (i.e., how their performance compares with their peers) as a means to judge the quality of their performance than are children who work under cooperative or individualistic goal structures. This theory may be especially relevant in the athletic setting where competition is such a salient issue. If a coach's praise and criticism are primarily contingent on performance *outcome* (i.e., winning or losing) rather than the *quality* of the performance itself, then the child may also learn to adopt peer comparison as the primary mode of competence judgment (e.g., "I am good at an activity only if I am a winner"). If, however, the coach's praise and criticism of a child's performance are based on other criteria such as degree of performance improvement or the quality of the skill technique regardless of the outcome, then the child may also learn to use such internal criteria in evaluating his or her competence (e.g., "I am good at an activity if I am getting better"). The criteria a coach or teacher uses to evaluate the child's performance may be especially important during the elementary school years (ages 6 to 12) because the developmental research indicates that peer comparison is a most salient source of information for children during this age range (Horn & Hasbrook, 1986). Coaches and teachers should use their evaluative feedback, then, to help children develop a more balanced perspective of self-assessment by emphasizing additional or alternative standards of success and failure.

In summary, the available research and theories do suggest that the praise and criticism given to children in an achievement setting influence their psychological growth. In particular, the contingency with which such feedback is given seems to provide children with information concerning (a) their competence, (b) the standard of performance they are expected to reach, and (c) the criteria by which their competence will be evaluated.

## Frequency and Contingency of Skill-Relevant Feedback

As discussed in the previous section, the evaluative nature of adults' feedback appears to be one factor that affects children's psychological growth. In this section, we will examine more closely the *informational* content of adults' feedback, particularly as that feedback is given in response to children's performance errors.

Within the last several years, considerable evidence has been accumulated to suggest that locus or perception of performance control is an important construct in explaining differences between children in their achievement behavior. In particular, an *internal* perception of control (i.e., a strong belief that performance outcomes are under the individual's own control) has been linked with many other positive psychological characteristics, including self-confidence, perceived competence, and intrinsic motivation (Harter & Connell, 1982; Stipek & Weisz, 1981; Wang, 1983). Internal perceived performance control has also been associated with a number of desirable achievement behaviors, such as persistence, task motivation, and high expectancy for success (Diener & Dweck, 1978, 1980; Gordon, Jones, & Short, 1977). Because children with an internal perception or locus of control truly believe that they can control their performance in an achievement activity, they are confident that they can achieve success through continued effort and practice or through the application of appropriate performance strategies. Thus, they are intrinsically motivated to pursue success in that domain. In contrast, children who feel that they have very little personal control of their performance outcome in an achievement domain exhibit little motivation to pursue success in that activity.

Based on this demonstrated association between children's perceptions of control and their subsequent achievement behavior, a number of researchers have recently conducted laboratory and field studies to examine how children's control perceptions can be facilitated in academic settings. The results of this research have demonstrated that certain instructional techniques such as individualized goal-setting procedures, self-monitoring training, and self-management training can be used to increase perceived performance control in children (Bandura & Schunk, 1981; McCombs, 1984; Wang, 1983).

Not surprisingly, evidence indicates that children's beliefs concerning their ability to control their performance are affected by the feedback they receive from adults in response to their performance. In particular, adults' responses to a child's performance failure may be most salient. Clifford (1984) recently presented a theory of "constructive failure" that argues that failure experiences in achievement contexts can be rendered nonaversive and even facilitative of future performance and motivation by teaching children to assume a problem-solving attitude in response to a performance error (e.g., "What did I do wrong? What can I do to improve my performance next time?"). From a locus-of-control perspective, the primary justification for this problem-solving attitude is based on the premise that a constructive analysis of a performance error will encourage children to believe that they can control the outcome of future performance attempts. However, two other lines of research also support the value of this approach. First, recent developments in the test anxiety literature suggest that a child whose attention is focused on task-analytic thoughts may be less apt to experience the more negative emotional and affective responses to failure (e.g., anxiety, shame, self-denigration, etc.) (Dusek, 1980; Fox & Houston, 1983; Wine, 1982). Second, a postfailure problem-solving attitude also induces the use of task-relevant self-talk, a cognitive strategy that has been associated with effective academic performance (Diener & Dweck, 1978, 1980) and enhanced motor skill performance (see review by Rushall, 1984).

To encourage children to develop such constructive, task-analytic cognitions and thus to bring their performance under their own control, several researchers have successfully employed cognitive modeling techniques (e.g., Meichenbaum & Goodman, 1971; Schunk, 1981). Under these types of programs a child is first exposed to an adult model who demonstrates the use of task-relevant and analytic thoughts during performance and who verbalizes his or her ability to control the performance outcome. Then, the child's use of these strategies is prompted during his or her own subsequent performance, with the ultimate intention of teaching the child to initiate such self-talk spontaneously. As Diener and Dweck (1978, 1980) have found, children who do respond to a performance error with task-analytic thoughts are also less apt even to define an "error" that occurs during an on-going performance as a failure but simply perceive it as a cue to initiate a different performance strategy and/or to try harder (e.g., "I need to concentrate harder"). In contrast, children who do not utilize such cognitive strategies perceive their "error" to indicate their lack of competence and inability to control future performance. These cognitive differences between children are clearly reflected in their subsequent performance and behavior. Children who employ task-relevant cognitions following a performance error also subsequently exhibit increased effort and improved performance, whereas children who respond to failure with non-task-relevant cognitions show impaired performance and lack of persistence, presumably because they feel unable to control performance outcomes.

The cumulative results of this research suggest that the most effective response a coach, teacher, or parent could make following a child's performance error would be to provide encouraging and skill-relevant corrective information (e.g., "Good try, Sally, but your initial step was too short; we'll keep working on it"). In fact, the value of this type of mistake-contingent response has already been demonstrated in the athletic setting via a series of well-designed studies conducted by Smith and Smoll and their associates (Smith et al., 1979; Smith et al., 1983; Smoll et al., 1978). In the first of these process-product studies (Smoll et al., 1978), the coaching behaviors of 51 Little League coaches were observed and recorded over the course of an entire playing season. At postseason, the 542 male players, aged 8 to 15, of these coaches were interviewed and their attitudes toward their teammates, the sport, and their coaches were measured. Correlational data analyses revealed that a coaching behavior profile characterized by high frequencies of mistake-contingent instruction and encouragement and a generally supportive and instructive communication style was significantly and positively correlated with players' attraction to their coaches, the sport, and the team.

In Phase 2 of this project (Smith et al., 1979), an experimental approach was used to demonstrate that these "effective" behaviors could be taught to youth sport coaches. Furthermore, observational and psychological data collected during the subsequent season revealed that athletes who played for these trained coaches exhibited greater postseason enjoyment of their sport experience and rated their coaches higher in knowledge and teaching technique than did players of untrained coaches. Finally, children who played for the trained coaches evidenced significant increases in self-esteem from the previous year, whereas players of control coaches did not show comparable changes.

In a subsequent process-product study conducted in a youth sport basketball league (Smith et al., 1983), the effectiveness of mistake-contingent technical instruction was even more clearly demonstrated. This study indicated that the frequency with which coaches provided error-contingent corrective instruction was the coaching behavior that was most highly predictive of athletes' postseason attitudes toward the sport and their evaluation of their coach.

The results of the research cited in this section suggest that mistake-contingent corrective instruction may be a crucial correlate of effective teaching and coaching behavior. Given that performance failures in competitive athletic settings have the potential to induce negative self-perceptions and affect in children, obviously the coach's response to those failures may have significant impact. Certainly, as Clifford (1984) has contended, performance errors committed by children in achievement settings do not need to be perceived as negative events but can actually be used by adults to facilitate children's psychosocial growth.

## Attributional Feedback

In a recent paper, Weiner (1979) applied his attribution theory to the educational setting by suggesting that the attributions children make for their academic successes and failures directly affect several aspects of their subsequent behavior. First, attribution of an academic success or failure to an internal cause (ability, effort) maximizes children's affective reactions and feelings (e.g., pride, shame, satisfaction, guilt) concerning their performance, whereas attribution to an external cause (e.g., behavior of others, luck, task difficulty) minimizes such affective feelings. Second, ascription of a success or failure to a stable cause (e.g., ability or task difficulty) encourages an expectancy within children that the same outcome will occur in the future, whereas attribution of a performance outcome to an unstable cause (e.g., mood, effort, luck) provides no consistent information regarding future performance outcomes. Finally, the belief that a performance outcome is due to a controllable cause (e.g., effort) encourages persistence and motivation to engage in that academic activity in the future.

Recently, several writers (e.g., Brophy, 1983; Schunk, 1984) have extended Weiner's (1979) theory on classroom motivation to propose that children's attributions for their academic successes and failures may be affected by the direct or implicit attribution contained in their teacher's responses to their classroom performances. Despite the logic of this hypothesis, very few researchers have actually attempted to measure the attributional content in the feedback given by teachers or coaches in instructional situations. One set of researchers to do so was Dweck, Davidson, Nelson, and Enna (1978). They collected attributional data as part of a larger observational study designed to assess possible gender differences in the feedback received by boys and girls in elementary classrooms. Analysis of their attributional data showed that (a) teachers tended to use attributional statements primarily in response to student failures and (b) boys received significantly more attribution to lack of effort as an explanation for their failure than did the girls. Dweck et al. did not collect corresponding product measures in their observational study; therefore, they could not assess how such differential feedback affected children's performance or psychosocial responses. However, the authors drew upon previous research in the learned helpless literature to suggest that the type of feedback received by the girls in their sample may promote feelings of helplessness in regard to personal achievement competencies.

At this point, then, we certainly do not have an extensive data base concerning the effects of attributional feedback as it is exhibited in field settings. This lack of research interest is probably largely due to the dearth of valid and reliable instrumentation to measure attributional feedback in naturalistic situations. The initial attempts that have been made to collect such information as part of more extensive process-product research projects (e.g., Dweck et al., 1978; Horn, 1985b; Parsons et al., 1982) have provided some information concerning the frequency, distribution, and potential effects of teachers' and coaches' verbal attributions. However, the establishment of definitive information in this area of study will be dependent on the development of adequate instrumentation.

In contrast to the lack of field-based data, considerable evidence for the impact of attributional feedback has been obtained through experimental manipulation of such feedback (e.g., Andrews & Debus, 1978; Dweck, 1975; Miller, Brickman, & Bolen, 1975; Schunk, 1982, 1983). In an early laboratory training study,

Dweck (1975) demonstrated that learned helpless children could be trained to use lack-of-effort rather than lack-of-ability attributions as a response to a performance error. This "attribution retraining" treatment proved to be significantly more effective in alleviating children's performance decrements following failure than was a success-only treatment. Dweck concluded that attribution to lack of effort is an effective cognitive response to failure for children in academic settings.

In general, the value of effort attributions as an *adult* response to children's performance outcomes has been shown in several subsequent laboratory projects (Andrews & Debus, 1978; Miller et al., 1975; Schunk, 1982). Each of these studies demonstrated that the experimenter's use of personal effort attributions as an explanation for children's performances facilitated their future performance and their perceptions regarding their academic competencies. According to attribution theory, ascription of performance outcomes to effort should be effective because level of effort is under the individual's volitional control. If children believe that a performance outcome was due to their level of personal effort, presumably they should also perceive that future performance is under their own control.

Schunk (1984), Brophy (1983), and Clifford (1984), however, have all recently advised some caution in concluding that effort attributions are always most advisable. Schunk explicitly points to the developmental research that suggests that children's understanding of the various performance causes changes with age. Specifically, young children (a) do not comprehend the role of luck in determining performance outcome (Nicholls & Miller, 1985; Weisz, Yeates, Robertson, & Beckham, 1982) and (b) cannot differentiate between ability and effort as performance causes (Nicholls, 1978; Stipek, 1981). Thus, the adult's attribution of a young child's performance failure to lack of effort may be understood by the child to indicate low competence or ability, whereas effort attributions for successes may be very effective in connoting high ability. Around age 9, however, when children begin to differentiate cognitively between ability and effort as causes of performance outcomes, ability may become increasingly more salient as a desirable attribute to possess. Thus ability attributions for success may be more effective than effort. This age-differential reaction to effort and ability was demonstrated in two unrelated studies. Miller et al. (1975) found that ability and effort attributions were equally effective adult responses to second graders' successes; both responses enhanced the mathematical skills and self-esteem of the children. In contrast, Schunk (1983), working with third graders, found that ability attributions given after successful performances were significantly more effective in facilitating self-efficacy and math performance than were attributions for those successes to effort.

The effectiveness of particular adult attributions, then, may well be dependent on the child's age. More information is needed regarding both the developmental changes in children's understanding and interpretation of the various

performance causes and the corresponding effectiveness of the forms of attributional feedback for children of different ages.

As a final point in regard to effort attributions, we also need to keep in mind
that attribution of performance failures to the child's lack of effort may be effective only if the child is persuaded that he or she possesses the requisite skills
to ultimately achieve performance success. Schunk (1982) found that the use
of effort attributions for children's past successes was effective in promoting
children's math performance and academic self-efficacy. In contrast, attributional feedback that only implied the need to exert effort in the future (e.g.,
"You need to work harder") was ineffective. In the motor skill setting, simply
providing a child with effort attribution only (e.g., "You need to try harder")
as a response to a performance failure (e.g., striking out for the third time
in a baseball game) may be highly ineffective because the child sees no reason
to believe that he or she has the ability to succeed even with additional effort.
However, effort (or lack of practice) attributions for a performance error may
be effective *if* accompanied by corrective feedback that tells the child how he
or she can achieve performance success in the future (e.g., "You are striking
out because you are dropping your elbow. You need to spend more practice
time on the batting machine this week."). Thus, in motor skill contexts, attributions for performance errors to the child's lack of experience, lack of practice,
or incorrect skill technique may be more effective than simply attributing such
errors to his or her lack of effort.

The available research and theory discussed in this section suggest that the
direct or implicit attribution contained in the feedback given by adults affects
the child's own interpretation of such performance successes and failures. However, considerably more research is necessary to provide adequate information
regarding the specific forms of attributional feedback that will be most effective
across a wide range of ages and skill levels. The research conducted to date
suggests that this is a very rich area for future researchers interested in identifying the correlates of effective teaching and coaching behavior.

## INSTRUCTIONAL EFFECTIVENESS:
## SUMMARY AND FUTURE DIRECTIONS

On the basis of the information obtained from this review of the process-product
research, the behaviors exhibited by instructors in both academic and motor
skill instructional settings apparently can influence the course of children's
psychological growth. In particular, we have identified three components of
adult behavior that appear to be most crucial to the development of various
psychological characteristics in children. We must recognize, however, that the
effectiveness of particular adult responses within each behavioral category will
vary, to a certain extent, as a function of several contextual factors including

the child's age, gender, ethnic/socioeconomic background, and level of performance skill.

Of these contextual factors, the child's age is probably the most important.
As was already pointed out, research in developmental psychology has shown
that children's beliefs, perceptions, cognitions, and interpretations of their
performance and their capabilities change, both quantitatively and qualitatively,
with increasing age (cf Harter, 1981; Nicholls, 1978; Stipek, 1981). Thus the
adult behaviors that are most effective in enhancing children's psychological
growth will likely vary as a function of the child's age. Such age-related differences in the correlates of effective teaching have already been demonstrated with
regard to children's academic achievement (see review by Brophy & Evertson,
1978). Researchers in the educational domain have found that the instructional
behaviors that are most effective in promoting the academic achievement of
upper elementary and junior high children are not necessarily the same behaviors as those found to be effective in the early elementary grades. In regard to
children's psychosocial growth, as well, the findings discussed in the previous
sections regarding age differences in children's reactions to adults' praise and
criticism and adults' use of effort versus ability attributions provide evidence
that the child's age is an important factor to consider in the search for effective
teaching and coaching behavior.

In addition to age as a mediating factor, evidence has also been accumulated
to show that other contextual factors—such as the child's gender, socioeconomic
status, level of skill, and psychological profile (e.g., level of trait anxiety,
self-esteem, etc.)—will also influence the effectiveness or ineffectiveness of
certain adult behaviors (Brophy & Evertson, 1978; Peterson, 1977). The likely
possibility of such context-specificity with regard to the correlates of instructional effectiveness has led a number of writers (e.g., Gage, 1979; Medley,
1979) to suggest that the course of future research lies in the empirical investigation and replication of process-product relationships within specific contexts. In
support of this issue, Gage (1979) has theorized that the identification of effective
instructional behaviors will ultimately result in a hierarchical structure. At the
base of the structure will be those few general teaching behaviors that have been
found to be effective across all contextual situations. However, the next hierarchical level will contain those instructional behaviors identified as most effective in a more limited context (i.e., at a certain age level), and each succeeding
level will consist of those behaviors that have been identified as effective in
increasingly more specific situations. Obviously, the identification of such a
hierarchy will require considerable and continued empirical research.

As Gage (1979) himself has recognized, the work involved in establishing
such a hierarchy is formidable considering the variety of contextual factors
that may influence instructional effectiveness. Nowhere is this more true than
in the motor skill instructional setting where so far a very small research base
has been established. Locke (1977), in his commentary emphasizing the lack

of process-product research in the physical education domain, also recognized the monumental nature of the task to be accomplished. To make such work easier and less prone to trial-and-error influences, Locke suggested that physical educators and researchers explore the literature in such related areas as the sociology and psychology of learning to identify existing theories that may be used to guide process-product research in the motor skill domain. This theoretically guided approach to the study of teaching or coaching effectiveness seems a most logical and reasonable way to begin. This chapter was meant to provide such a theoretical framework. To that end, the relevant research from both the theoretical and empirically based literatures were examined for the purpose of identifying three categories of adult behavior that seem most important to children's psychological growth. These are offered with the recommendation that extensive and replicated process-product research in both laboratory and field settings be conducted using the three identified behavioral components as a guide to the measurement and analysis of instructional behavior.

As the review of the literature in this chapter has shown, much work still needs to be done in the motor skill domain with respect to teaching and coaching effectiveness. Given the demonstrated influence, however, of adult behavior on the psychological development of the child, such work should be well justified.

## REFERENCES

Ames, C., & Ames, R. (1984). Systems of student and teacher motivation: Toward a qualitative definition. *Journal of Educational Psychology, 76*, 535–556.

Anderson, R., Manoogian, S.T., & Reznick, J.S. (1976). The undermining and enhancing of intrinsic motivation in preschool children. *Journal of Personality and Social Psychology, 34*, 915–922.

Andrews, G., & Debus, R. (1978). Persistence and the causal perception of failure: Modifying cognitive attributions. *Journal of Educational Psychology, 70*, 154–166.

Bandura, A. (1977). Self-efficacy: Toward a unifying theory of behavioral change. *Psychological Review, 84*, 191–215.

Bandura, A., & Schunk, D. (1981). Cultivating competence, self-efficacy, and intrinsic interest through proximal self-motivation. *Journal of Personality and Social Psychology, 41*, 586–598.

Boggiano, A.K., & Ruble, D.N. (1979). Competence and the overjustification effect: A developmental study. *Journal of Personality and Social Psychology, 37*, 1462–1468.

Brookover, W., Schweitzer, J., Schneider, J., Beady, C., Flood, P., & Wisenbaker, J. (1978). Elementary school social climate and school achievement. *American Educational Research Journal,* **15**, 301–318.

Brophy, J. (1981). Teacher praise: A functional analysis. *Review of Educational Research,* **51**, 5–32.

Brophy, J. (1983). Conceptualizing student motivation. *Educational Psychologist,* **18**, 200–215.

Brophy, J., & Evertson, C. (1976). *Learning from teaching: A developmental perspective.* Boston: Allyn & Bacon.

Brophy, J., & Evertson, C. (1978). Context variables in teaching. *Educational Psychologist,* **12**, 310–316.

Brophy, J., & Good, T. (1974). *Teacher-student relationships: Causes and consequences.* New York: Holt, Rinehart, & Winston.

Clifford, M. (1984). Thoughts on a theory of constructive failure. *Educational Psychologist,* **19**, 108–120.

Coakley, J.J. (1987). Children and the sport socialization process. In D. Gould & M.R. Weiss (Eds.), *Advances in pediatric sport sciences: Vol. 2. Behavioral issues* (pp. 43–60). Champaign, IL: Human Kinetics.

Cooper, H., & Good, T. (1983). *Pygmalion grows up: Studies in the expectation communication process.* New York: Longman.

Deci, E.L., & Ryan, R.M. (1985). *Intrinsic motivation and self-determination in human behavior.* New York: Plenum.

Diener, C., & Dweck, C. (1978). An analysis of learned helplessness: Continuous changes in performance, strategy, and achievement cognitions following failure. *Journal of Personality and Social Psychology,* **36**, 451–462.

Diener, C., & Dweck, C. (1980). An analysis of learned helplessness: II. The processing of success. *Journal of Personality and Social Psychology,* **39**, 940–952.

Dusek, J.B. (1980). The development of test anxiety in children. In I.G. Sarason (Ed.), *Test anxiety: Theory, research, and applications* (pp. 87–110). Hillsdale, NJ: Erlbaum.

Dweck, C. (1975). The role of expectations and attributions in the alleviation of learned helplessness. *Journal of Personality and Social Psychology,* **31**, 674–685.

Dweck, C., Davidson, W., Nelson, S., & Enna, B. (1978). Sex differences in learned helplessness: II. The contingencies of evaluative feedback in the classroom and III. An experimental analysis. *Developmental Psychology,* **14**, 268–276.

Fox, J., & Houston, B. (1983). Distinguishing between cognitive and somatic trait and state anxiety in children. *Journal of Personality and Social Psychology, 45*, 862–870.

Gage, N. (1979). The generality of dimensions of teaching. In P.L. Peterson & H.J. Walberg (Eds.), *Research on teaching: Concepts, findings, and implications* (pp. 264–288). Berkeley, CA: McCutchan.

Good, T., Ebmeier, H., & Beckerman, T. (1978). Teaching mathematics in high and low SES classrooms: An empirical comparison. *Journal of Teacher Education, 29*, 85–90.

Gordon, D., Jones, R., & Short, N. (1977). Task persistence and locus of control in elementary school children. *Child Development, 48*, 1716–1719.

Harter, S. (1981). A model of intrinsic mastery motivation in children: Individual differences and developmental change. In W.C. Collins (Ed.), *Minnesota Symposium on Child Psychology* (Vol. 14, pp. 215–254). Hillsdale, NJ: Erlbaum.

Harter, S., & Connell, J.P. (1982). A comparison of alternative models of the relationship between academic achievement and children's perceptions of competence, control, and motivational orientation. In J. Nicholls (Ed.), *The development of achievement-related cognitions and behaviors* (pp. 153–197). Greenwich, CT: JAI Press.

Horn, T.S. (1985a). Coaches' feedback and changes in children's perceptions of their physical competence. *Journal of Educational Psychologist, 77*, 174–186.

Horn, T.S. (1985b, April). *Coaches' attributional feedback: Effects on the self-perceptions of junior high female athletes*. Paper presented at the meeting of the American Alliance for Health, Physical Education, Recreation, and Dance, Atlanta, GA.

Horn, T.S., & Hasbrook, C. (1986). Informational components influencing children's perceptions of their physical competence. In M. Weiss & D. Gould (Eds.), *Sport for children and youths* (pp. 81–88). Champaign, IL: Human Kinetics.

Kleinfeld, J. (1975). Effective teachers of Eskimo and Indian students. *School Review, 83*, 301–344.

Krohne, H.W. (1980). Parental child-rearing behavior and the development of anxiety and coping strategies in children. In I.G. Sarazon & C.D. Spielberger (Eds.), *Stress and anxiety* (Vol. 7, pp. 233–245). Washington, DC: Hemisphere.

Locke, L. (1977). Research on teaching physical education: New hope for a dismal science. *Quest, 28*, 2–16.

Martin, J., Veldman, D., & Anderson, L.M. (1980). Within-class relationships between student achievement and teacher behaviors. *American Educational Research Journal, 17*, 479–490.

McCombs, B. (1984). Processes and skills underlying continuing intrinsic motivation to learn: Toward a definition of motivational skills training interventions. *Educational Psychologist, 19*, 199–218.

Medley, D.M. (1979). The effectiveness of teachers. In P.L. Peterson & H.J. Walberg (Eds.), *Research on teaching: Concepts, findings, & implications* (pp. 11–27). Berkeley, CA: McCutchan.

Meichenbaum, D., & Goodman, J. (1971). Training impulsive children to talk to themselves: A means of developing self-control. *Journal of Abnormal Psychology, 77*, 115–126.

Meyer, W., Bachmann, M., Biermann, U., Hempelmann, M., Ploger, F., & Spiller, H. (1979). The informational value of evaluative behavior: Influences of praise and blame on perceptions of ability. *Journal of Educational Psychology, 71*, 259–268.

Meyer, W., Mittag, W., & Engler, U. (1985). *"Paradoxical" effects of praise and blame on perceived ability and affect.* Unpublished manuscript, University of Bielefeld, West Germany.

Miller, R., Brickman, P., & Bolen, D. (1975). Attribution versus persuasion as a means for modifying behavior. *Journal of Personality and Social Psychology, 31*, 430–441.

Nicholls, J. (1978). The development of the concepts of effort and ability, perception of academic attainment, and the understanding that difficult tasks require more ability. *Child Development, 49*, 800–814.

Nicholls, J., & Miller, A. (1985). Differentiation of the concepts of luck and skill. *Developmental Psychology, 21*, 76–82.

Parsons, J.E., Kaczala, C.M., & Meece, J.L. (1982). Socialization of achievement attitudes and beliefs: Classroom influences. *Child Development, 53*, 322–339.

Passer, M. (1983). Fear of failure, fear of evaluation, perceived competence, and self-esteem in competitive trait anxious children. *Journal of Sport Psychology, 5*, 172–188.

Peterson, P. (1977). Interactive effects of student anxiety, achievement orientation, and teacher behavior on student achievement and attitude. *Journal of Educational Psychology, 69*, 779–792.

Pittman, T.S., Davey, M.E., Alafat, K.A., Wetherill, K.V., & Kramer, N.A. (1980). Informational versus controlling verbal rewards. *Personality and Social Psychology Bulletin, 6*, 228–233.

Rushall, B. (1984). The content of competition thinking. In W. Straub & J. Williams (Eds.), *Cognitive sport psychology* (pp. 51–62). Lansing, NY: Sport Science Associates.

Ryan, R. (1982). Control and information in the intrapersonal sphere: An extension of cognitive evaluation theory. *Journal of Personality and Social Psychology,* **43**, 450–461.

Schunk, D. (1981). Modeling and attributional effects on children's achievement: A self-efficacy analysis. *Journal of Educational Psychology,* **73**, 93–105.

Schunk, D. (1982). Effects of effort attributional feedback on children's perceived self-efficacy and achievement. *Journal of Educational Psychology,* **74**, 548–556.

Schunk, D. (1983). Ability versus effort attributional feedback: Differential effects on self-efficacy and achievement. *Journal of Educational Psychology,* **75**, 848–856.

Schunk, D. (1984). Self-efficacy perspective on achievement behavior. *Educational Psychologist,* **19**, 48–58.

Smith, R.E., Smoll, F.L., & Curtis, B. (1979). Coach effectiveness training: A cognitive-behavioral approach to enhancing relationship skills in youth sport coaches. *Journal of Sport Psychology,* **1**, 59–75.

Smith, R., Zane, N., Smoll, F., & Coppel, D. (1983). Behavioral assessment in youth sports: Coaching behaviors and children's attitudes. *Medicine and Science in Sports and Exercise,* **15**, 208–214.

Smoll, F.L., Smith, R.E., Curtis, B., & Hunt, E. (1978). Toward a mediational model of coach-player relationships. *Research Quarterly,* **49**, 528–541.

Solomon, D., & Kendall, A. (1976). Individual characteristics and children's performance in "open" and "traditional" classroom settings. *Journal of Educational Psychology,* **68**, 613–625.

Stipek, D. (1981). Children's perceptions of their own and their classmates ability. *Journal of Educational Psychology,* **73**, 404–410.

Stipek, D., & Weisz, J. (1981). Perceived personal control and academic achievement. *Review of Educational Research,* **51**, 101–137.

Vallerand, R.J., & Reid, G. (1984). On the causal effects of perceived competence on intrinsic motivation: A test of cognitive evaluation theory. *Journal of Sport Psychology,* **6**, 94–102.

Wang, M. (1983). Development and consequences of students' sense of personal control. In J.M. Levine & M.C. Wang (Eds.), *Teacher and student perceptions: Implications for learning* (pp. 213–247). Hillsdale, NJ: Erlbaum.

Weiner, B. (1979). A theory of motivation for some classroom experiences. *Journal of Educational Psychology, 71*, 3–25.

Weinstein, R. (1976). Reading group membership in first grade: Teacher behaviors and pupil experience over time. *Journal of Educational Psychology, 68*, 103–116.

Weisz, J., Yeates, K., Robertson, D., & Beckham, J. (1982). Perceived contingency of skill and chance events: A developmental analysis. *Developmental Psychology, 18*, 898–905.

Wine, J. (1982). Evaluation anxiety: A cognitive-attentional construct. In H.W. Krohne & L. Laux (Eds.), *Achievement, stress, & anxiety* (pp. 207–219). Washington, DC: Hemisphere.

# 7

# Moral Growth Through Physical Activity: A Structural/Developmental Approach

**Brenda Jo Bredemeier**
**David L. Shields**

As children play, they are not only physical actors but also moral agents. Game and sport activity provides children with a context of interpersonal action that is shaped by shared norms and reciprocal moral expectations. In this chapter, we seek to shed some light on this often neglected dimension of pediatric sport science, emphasizing a structural/developmental interpretation of morality.

Our chapter opens with a discussion of the emergence of two theoretical approaches to moral development, internalization and structural development. This discussion highlights the two most important investigations of moral development conducted during the first half of this century, both of which employed physical activity as a context for the exploration of children's morality. We then turn to an exploration of current theory, elaborating two structural developmental models of moral growth. The third section presents a review of internalization and structural/developmental literature, focusing on selected issues pertinent to the moral development of young sport participants. Finally, we offer three general recommendations for constructing sport experiences designed to promote children's moral growth.

## MORAL GROWTH: INTERNALIZATION OR STRUCTURAL DEVELOPMENT?

Two major perspectives on moral development may be traced from the present back to the 1920s. One perspective is advocated by internalization theorists who view moral development as the learning of socially acceptable behavior through transmitted values. Both psychoanalytic and social learning theorists fall into this category, equating moral development with the child's progressive internalization of social regulations. The theorists diverge, however, in their understanding of the internalization process. Whereas psychoanalytic theory highlights psychodynamic processes tied to the id, ego, and superego, social learning theory points to the role of socializing agents in transmitting cultural norms.

The second major moral development perspective encompasses structural/ developmentalists' views. These theorists maintain that moral growth results from an interaction between (a) the individual's innate tendency to organize experience into coherent patterns of meaningful interpretation and (b) environmental experiences that provide information about social reality. Thus, moral development is seen as a process of reorganizing and transforming the underlying structure of one's reasoning.

These two perspectives may be more clearly illustrated by juxtaposing two classic studies of children's morality. The work of Hartshorne and May (1928; Hartshorne, May, & Maller, 1929; Hartshorne, May, & Shuttleworth, 1930) and, in particular, a study designed to investigate children's cheating in athletic contests will represent the internalization perspective. It will be contrasted with Piaget's (1932) structural/developmental account of children's understanding and practice of rules in the game of marbles.

In their first volume of *Studies in the Nature of Character*, Hartshorne and May (1928) described a study in which a school athletic contest was employed to assess girls' and boys' honesty. The researchers considered the virtue of honesty to be one of the socially valued traits that comprise mature moral character. The school athletic contest was one of 33 different studies designed to assess three types of deceitful conduct: cheating, lying, and stealing.

Contest participants included 2,175 girls and boys in Grades 4 through 10. The students were told that their school was holding a "physical ability contest" and that specific handicaps had been arranged so that all had a chance to win a badge in each of four events: grip strength, lung capacity, pull-ups, and the standing long jump.

For each of the four events, an examiner first demonstrated the task and offered careful instruction then directed the student to do a specific number of practice trials. After coaching and urging the student to achieve a good practice trial score, the examiner instructed the student to perform a specified number of contest trials when alone. Finally, the student was requested to report the best contest trial performance so that the score could be compared to those of her or his competitors. If the student reported any contest score that was higher than the best practice score, the researchers assumed that deception had taken place.

From a vantage point improved by 50 years of development in the social sciences, we may question some of the assumptions in Hartshorne and May's design and methodology. Contemporary sport psychologists might contend, for example, that performing alone for the contest may have been more conducive to a good performance than performing practice trials in the presence of the examiner. Moral development researchers might argue that tests such as the athletic contest actually tap children's conceptualizations of social convention rather than morality (Turiel, 1983). Although Hartshorne and May's elaborate series of investigations contained methodological flaws, investigators still generally agree with many of their specific findings about the nature of moral traits like honesty (Blasi, 1980).

When Hartshorne and May compared the athletic contest results with data from other behavioral measures of honesty, they found only low correlations between tests. They concluded that little evidence existed that the general trait of honesty is present within individuals and proposed the "doctrine of specificity." Virtues like honesty and dishonesty, they wrote, should not be viewed as unified character traits but as specific behaviors that correspond to specific life situations. If an individual demonstrates consistent behavior in separate situations, it is because the situations have similar features. Consistency, Hartshorne and May maintained, may be found across certain life situations but not within individuals.

From a number of studies, Hartshorne and May also concluded that moral thought and moral action have little relation to each other. A child who said, for example, that cheating is wrong was no more likely to refrain from cheating than a child who approved of cheating. Apparently, Hartshorne and May concluded, "moral knowledge" has little relation to moral action.

Whereas Hartshorne and May began their studies by defining what constitutes right moral action and then designed tests to see whether children behaved as the investigators thought they should, Piaget (1932) took a different approach. A brief sketch of Piaget's general perspective on the development of knowledge will help us understand his approach to moral reasoning and behavior.

Prior to Piaget, knowledge was generally assessed through the employment of IQ tests designed to measure the quantity of information that a person had amassed. The assumption was that a child was a miniature adult, differing from the latter only in that the child possessed less information. What interested Piaget, however, were the "wrong" answers that children gave to questions. Through probing children's reasoning for giving wrong answers, Piaget soon found that children were not making random errors; rather, their "mistakes" reflected a coherent pattern of cognition. The principles by which children organized their experience, he discovered, were different from those used by adults. In other words, children not only have less information, they also understand and organize their knowledge differently.

This insight led to a different approach to the question of the relationship between thought and action. IQ tests, much like the Hartshorne and May honesty tests, were designed to determine how closely children's behavior (responses to test questions) corresponded with what adults consider the right responses. For Piaget the question became, In what way does children's behavior reflect the organization of their thought?

Piaget distinguished between the *structure* of mental functioning and the *content* of one's beliefs, knowledge, and action. Content includes the discreet bits of information that a person knows and the particular behavioral choices a person makes. Cognitive structure, on the other hand, is comprised of those rules and principles of mental functioning that give coherence to thinking. Corresponding to the content-structure distinction are two dimensions of development. As children mature, they gain quantitatively in the amount of information they know and, in addition, the organizing principles of their cognitive processes undergo qualitative transformations.

Piaget's studies led him to conclude that children's thought evolves through an invariant series of stages. Each succeeding stage of development represents a qualitatively new way of organizing information. Piaget's view is referred to as a structural/developmental, or more specifically, a cognitive/developmental perspective. From this viewpoint, children's behavior is seen to reflect the patterning of their thought as it is engaged by experiences in the environment. Thus, behavior is mediated by an interaction between the active structuring mind and environmental stimuli.

The understanding of morality as a structural/developmental construct originated with Piaget's observation of Swiss children's play in the microcosm of the common Geneva street game of marbles (Piaget, 1932). From his observations and probing questions, Piaget concluded that two major stages are present in children's moral development. For a child at the "heteronomous stage," rules are seen as rigid, unalterable dictates, sacred because they come from the world of adults. The irony is that children at this stage rarely conform to the rules! Piaget's interpretation of this paradoxical observation was that even though children behave idiosyncratically, they believe that their behavior conforms to the rules. What may appear to adults as inconsistent is consistent from the child's viewpoint because of the child's egocentric way of organizing information.

As the child progresses to the "autonomous" stage of morality, an orientation toward cooperation with peers supercedes conformity to adult constraint. Although the child now views rules as more flexible and subject to change, he or she follows them more rigidly. Again, the apparent inconsistency is consistent from the child's viewpoint. Although rules are themselves viewed as more flexible, a less egocentric viewpoint allows the child to conform to the social norms of his or her peers.

Piaget's work differed from that of Hartshorne and May in three important respects. First, Hartshorne and May equated morality with a set of arbitrarily selected character traits that adult society values. In contrast, Piaget conceived of morality as equivalent to the child's growing understanding of the nature of social regulation. Second, Hartshorne and May believed that moral behavior is determined primarily by the environment. Piaget believed that the child's constructions of social reality are as important as the environmental constraints. Finally, Hartshorne and May looked for thought-action consistency in terms of a direct correlation between moral beliefs and moral action. Piaget contended that the route from thought to action is not so direct. Moral beliefs are items of moral content and before one can understand the relation between moral thought and moral action, one must move beneath an analysis of content to an investigation of the underlying structure. One can then look for consistency between thought structure organization and patterns of behavior.

## CONTEMPORARY MORAL DEVELOPMENT THEORY

Modern sport psychology has been influenced primarily by social learning theorists. These scientists define morality as prosocial behavior and conceive of it as a learned behavior influenced primarily by the modeling and reinforcement of significant others. Although self-regulatory mechanisms may be viewed as important determinants, these, too, are said to originate ultimately from an internalization of environmental experiences. In an effort to maintain scientific rigor, researchers often define the internal organization of thought, which is not directly observable, as outside the realm of investigation.

Social learning theorists have contributed significantly to our understanding of moral action. We believe, however, that if sport psychology is to continue to develop its theoretical base for investigating the moral dimensions of play, games, and sport, insights from structural developmental psychologists need to be utilized also. In this section, we review two important contemporary advocates of this approach.

### Kohlberg's Cognitive Theory

Piaget's work on morality was like a seed with a long germination period and it lay dormant in American soil until rediscovered by Lawrence Kohlberg in the late 1950s. Kohlberg shared Piaget's cognitive/developmental perspective but expanded the scope of Piaget's inquiry and thoroughly revised his stages of moral development.

Kohlberg's (1981, 1984) method of investigation involved interviewing people about hypothetical situations of moral conflict between two or more basic moral values (e.g., honesty and loyalty). Unlike Hartshorne and May, Kohlberg was not trying to measure the virtues of honesty and loyalty. Rather, he was interested in the pattern of reasoning people use to decide which value is most important in a given situation. Thus, being honest in one situation and not honest in another situation may not necessarily reflect inconsistency. The individual may be perfectly consistent in following a logic of when to be honest and when not to be.

By posing hypothetical dilemmas and probing people's reasoning about what the main character in the story should do—and more importantly, *why* she or he should do it—Kohlberg uncovered what he believes to be six universal stages of moral development. The six stages are divided into three levels, each of which denotes a significant expansion of moral conceptualizations from an ego-centric through a societal to a universal moral perspective. A person reasoning at the preconventional level is unconcerned with the effects of actions on broader social groups and is primarily interested in his or her own welfare. At the conventional level, social norms and expectations are central considerations in resolving moral dilemmas. Finally, for those who achieve postconventional or principled reasoning, morality is organized by a concern for universal principles that are not restricted by the limitations of a particular culture. Each stage of moral development is summarized in Table 1.

Kohlberg posits that each successive stage of development represents a more adequate understanding of justice, the defining concept of morality. Each higher stage, he maintains, is "better" than lower stages both psychologically, in that it is more inclusive and logically consistent, and philosophically, in that it comes closer to meeting formal criteria for adequacy, such as prescriptivity and universalizability. Kohlberg also maintains that all people pass through the same sequence of stages, though culture will affect the content of moral beliefs, the rate of stage progression, and the likelihood of ever reaching the postconventional level.

Although Kohlberg's work represents a major advance in the structural/developmental study of morality, it has been criticized on a number of grounds. Carol Gilligan (1982), for example, has maintained that the concept of justice does not adequately address the theme of care that is central in women's moral reasoning. Several critics have attacked the formalism of Kohlberg's ethics (Alston, 1971; Aron, 1977; Munsey, 1980). Similarly, others have charged that Kohlberg's theory is ethnocentric and does not reflect universal moral structures (Shweder, 1982; Simpson, 1974; Sullivan, 1977). Still others have suggested that the emotional dimensions involved in moral decision making

to be restored. Moral dialogue must occur to recreate the balance and reach common understanding and agreement, so that social exchange can continue and life can go on.

Sport is full of implicit moral balances. Informal agreements or balances exist between a coach and players about such issues as the length and demands of practice; special favors that may be received for performance; and who will play, for how long, and under what conditions. Balances also exist between team members regarding who has what rights and what responsibilities. For example, among some teams, more skilled players may be expected to assist less skilled players in the development of their capabilities. Balances are also achieved between teams as they negotiate (most often nonverbally) about what kinds of behaviors are acceptable in competitive contexts and under what conditions. Many of the unspoken rules of the game come under this heading.

The qualitative uniqueness of every moral situation is an issue to which Haan's model of interactional morality is responsive. Moral decisions, for Haan, must reflect the intricacies of human interaction. Abstract ethical principles—and the universalizable decisions to which they lead—do not adequately respond to the nature of our moral life. As an alternative to deductive moral reasoning that operates from pre-existing principles, Haan offers a model of inductive moral reasoning that describes people's continual reconstruction of moral meaning.

**The nature of moral truth**. Every moral theory must specify its moral grounds. Kohlberg has done this in terms of the principle of justice. Haan argues that an abstract principle cannot be employed to adequately resolve the multitude of intricately nuanced decisions that must be made in everyday life. Consequently, rather than focusing on principles for determining right answers to moral problems, Haan specifies her moral grounds in terms of procedures. The moral dialogue itself must meet four conditions if it is to truly be a *moral* dialogue.

First, a valid moral dialogue must seek consensus. All parties must accept the solution as the best that can be achieved given the limitations of the situation and the unique characteristics of the discussants. All persons hold power of veto, and any use of force to gain a resolution automatically invalidates the conclusions. Second, participants must have equal opportunity to influence the conclusions. Any restrictions on the freedom to participate equally in moral exchange inevitably results in moral distortions. Third, all participants must have equal access to information. Finally, valid moral dialogues only take place when participants are mindful of their future lives together. When dialogue is not rooted in a recognition of interdependency, it drifts easily into abstract formulations that are no longer grounded in the concrete construction of moral balance.

In everyday life, we rarely, if ever, fully meet the conditions for a truth-identifying moral dialogue. Seldom do all parties have full access to relevant information, and decisions are usually not based on completely nondominated discussion. Though the moral balances we construct are less than perfect, we must nonetheless reflect on the conditions for ideal moral dialogue so that we can approximate them and so that our imperfect moral agreements will not be reified into moral truth.

**Moral development**. The ability to participate in truth-identifying moral dialogues is not innate. Haan's research suggests that as children mature, their ability to engage in sound moral dialogue evolves through a series of levels. She has identified five levels; each successive level represents a more adequate ability to participate in the construction of moral balance and a more accurate understanding of the truth-identifying procedures of moral negotiation. Brief summaries of each level are presented in Table 2.

### Table 2

### Levels of Interactional Morality

---

#### Assimilation phase

*Level 1: Power balancing.* The person is unable to sustain a view of others' interest apart from self-interest and vacillates between compliance with others when forced and thwarting others when able to do so. Balances reflect self-interest except for situations where the self is indifferent or forced to compromise.

*Level 2: Egocentric balancing.* The person is able to differentiate others' interests from self-interest but does not understand that both may coincide in a mutual interest. People are viewed as essentially self-interested and out for their own good. To get what the self wants, trade-offs or compromises are made.

#### Accommodation phase

*Level 3: Harmony balancing.* The person differentiates others' interest from self-interest but assumes that a harmony of these interests can be found by giving to others since most people are believed to possess altruistic motives. Balances are sought that rest on the good faith of all. People of bad faith are considered odd and dismissed from moral consideration.

*Level 4: Common interest balancing.* The person differentiates all parties' self-interests from the common interest of the group. Balances of compromise are sought that conform to the system-maintenance requirements of the group. Because the moral culpability of all is recognized, externally regulated patterns of exchange are sought that benefit all while limiting personal vulnerability.

#### Equilibration phase

*Level 5: Mutual interest balancing.* The person coordinates all parties' self-interests and the common interest of the group in a search for a situationally specific moral balance that will optimize everyone's interest. In such a search, the person recognizes the need to consider the specific values and desires, strengths and vulnerabilities, of the parties involved. Solutions may achieve harmony of interests or may represent compromises of interest, whatever the particularities of the situation and participants allow.

---

*Note.* Adapted from Shields, 1986.

## CHILDREN'S SPORT EXPERIENCE
## AND MORAL DEVELOPMENT

In reviewing selected dimensions of the empirical research into children's moral experience of sport, dividing the literature into two categories is helpful: (a) internalization and (b) structural/developmental research.

### Internalization Research

Internalization theorists tend to employ a "bag-of-virtues" approach to research, operationalizing morality in terms of selected character traits or virtues. Social scientists using this approach to investigate young sport participants' moral growth have focused on personality characteristics, value orientations, and prosocial behavior.

**Personality characteristics.** Efforts to assess, and thus learn to effectively promote, the development of desired personality characteristics among children involved in physical activity began in the 1930s (McCloy, 1930) and can be illustrated by a study conducted by Blanchard (1946). Investigating a bag of virtues that included such interpersonal qualities as cooperation, self-control, and sociability, Blanchard found that for a sample population of 8th through 11th graders, increases in these character traits were associated with participation in physical education classes. The findings were significantly stronger for girls than for boys.

The Blanchard investigation suffered from two shortcomings that characterize much of the internalization literature. First, the logic behind the selection of traits for study was simply a logic of preference; no clear theoretical rationale justified the selection of cooperation, self-control, and sociability as dependent variables. Conclusions drawn from such studies are frequently misleading; in this case, for example, Blanchard contended that boys had benefited less than girls from the physical education program. Because Blanchard, a female researcher, investigated interpersonal qualities congruent with the female gender role, it is not suprising that it was the female subjects who showed greater gains. Second, Blanchard succumbed to a classic interpretation error in assuming that the physical education program *caused* the observed changes. Her design did not control for the influence of other factors, such as maturation or nonphysical education experiences; thus, causal relations were not adequately determined.

**Value orientations.** Several researchers have examined participants' value orientations toward sport, chronicling the development of the relative significance of intrasport values. Webb (1969) initiated this research, demonstrating with cross-sectional data that as age and sport experience increase a progressive change in value orientations occurs. A "play orientation," consisting of a value hierarchy of fairness, skill, and success in that order, becomes increasingly subordinated to a "professional orientation" in which success is most valued and fairness least. The professionalization of values has been found to vary, not only with age and sport experience but also with gender: Males consistently score higher on professionalization than females (Loy, 1975; Maloney & Petrie, 1974; Mantel & Velden, 1974; Petrie, 1971; Sage, 1980; Webb, 1969). As children become older and more involved in organized sport, they tend to move from a play to a professional orientation.

The professionalization studies also contain several weaknesses in that they focus on changes in content, not structure. As children mature, their conceptualizations evolve. Thus, having people rate fairness, skill, and success in hierarchical order tells us little because the meaning of the concepts themselves does not remain constant from one age to another. Are the observed changes due to structural changes in valuing, or do they reflect a constant value toward conformity to social expectations, expectations which vary from less competitive to more elite sports? Finally, these studies, by design, do not shed light on how the "value changes" impact on people's thinking and behavior outside the realm of sport.

**Prosocial behavior.** A third set of internalization studies has been conducted by social learning theorists interested in the effects of sport on the development of children's prosocial behavior. These theorists operationalize morality in terms of objectively observable behaviors, such as sharing, taking turns, and cooperation with peers. Kleiber and Roberts (1981) used this model to investigate the influence of participation in sport competition on cooperation and altruism. Fourth- and fifth-grade children were randomly assigned to a control or experimental group; the experimental group competed in a kickball tournament during a 20-minute recess period for 8 days. Before and after the tournament, prosocial behaviors were assessed using a paper-and-pencil scale. Results indicated that boys in the experimental group demonstrated significantly less altruistic behavior after the tournament as compared to boys in the control group. The investigators interpreted these results as tentative support for the view that sport competition can have a negative impact on character development. These results, however, should be viewed, as the authors themselves suggest, with considerable caution because only a single test of altruism was used, and altruism itself is only a single dimension of morality. Furthermore, the intervention was of short duration, and the findings were not consistent across sex.

Orlick (1981) also employed a prosocial behavior approach to investigate the relative effects of 18-week traditional and cooperative games programs on the willingness of the 5-year-old participants to share. Children took part in either a traditional or cooperative games program offered by one of two participating schools; program activity levels and physical demands were matched as far as possible. Willingness to share was assessed using a candy-sharing task. Orlick found conflicting results in that (a) the cooperative games participants in one school showed a significant increase in willingness to share, whereas the other school's cooperative games participants showed no change; and (b) willingness to share significantly declined for children in one school's traditional program but did not change for children in the other school's traditional program. Although Orlick's study provides limited support for the relative merit of a cooperative games program, the study, like that of Kleiber and Roberts, is severely limited by the single dimension of morality investigated.

Finally, Giebink and McKenzie (1985) employed instructional strategies based on social learning theory to teach sportsmanship ("positive social interaction related to game play") to four boys. Intervention strategies included instructions and praise, modeling, and a point-reward system. Results indicated that all three strategies increased sportsmanship, but attempts to demonstrate participants' generalization to a recreation setting were unsuccessful. Weaknesses included the tiny sample and the purely behavioral assessment of sportsmanship. As other social scientists have suggested (Bredemeier & Shields, 1983; Figley, 1984), the rationale behind the choice of behavior determines the morality of the behavior.

Taken as a whole, these studies point to the need for a unified and theoretically grounded understanding of moral thought and action. This is what structural/developmental theorists seek to offer.

## Structural/Developmental Research

Structural/developmental theory has been employed only recently to investigate children's morality in a sport context. To date, investigators have been able to shed light on four major questions: Do children reason about moral issues in sport in the same way as they reason about moral issues in other life contexts? What is the relationship between sport participation and moral reasoning maturity? Is the moral reasoning maturity of a sport participant related to his or her behavioral tendencies? Finally, can moral growth be facilitated through sport experiences?

**Life-sport reasoning differences.** The question of children's context-specific moral reasoning grew out of a study indicating that high school and college athletes and nonathletes reason about moral issues in the context of sport differently than they reason about moral issues in other life settings (Bredemeier & Shields, 1984a). Reasoning about sport often reflects a more egocentric form of moral reasoning that Bredemeier and Shields (1986a) have termed "game reasoning." In a recent investigation, Bredemeier (in press-b) sought to determine when this divergence between life and sport reasoning begins to appear. A study of 110 preadolescents revealed that children 11 years old and younger did not demonstrate context-specific moral reasoning patterns. The 12- and 13-year-old children, however, reasoned at a significantly lower (more egocentric) level in response to the sport dilemmas as compared to general life dilemmas. Several explanations for these findings are possible. Interpretations could emphasize (a) the changing demands of sport as children mature; (b) advances in children's cognitive functioning, allowing for a clearer differentiation between life and sport contexts; or (c) development in general "life" moral reasoning toward a more altruistic perspective that may conflict with the norms of sport.

**Sport participation and moral reasoning maturity.** The question of the relationship between participation in sport and children's moral maturity was poignantly raised by evidence indicating that basketball players at the collegiate level are less mature in their moral reasoning than their nonathlete peers (Bredemeier & Shields, 1984b, 1986b; Hall, 1981). Extending this line of research to children, Bredemeier, Weiss, Shields, and Cooper (in press-b) studied the relationship between children's participation in high-, medium-, and low-contact youth sports and their moral reasoning maturity. The sample was comprised of 106 children in Grades 4 through 7 participating in a summer sport camp program. Results indicated that boys' participation in high-contact sports (e.g., football and ice hockey) and girls' participation in medium-contact sports (e.g., basketball and soccer, the roughest sports in which girls reported participating) were significantly correlated with less mature moral reasoning. No other participation-reasoning relationships were significant. These results may indicate that the meaning girls attach to their participation in medium-contact sports is similar to the meaning boys attach to participation in high-contact sports. A structural/developmental interpretation of these findings posits that moral reasoning maturity is not related to the sport structure in isolation; rather, reasoning maturity is related to an interaction between the sport structure and the interpretive framework of the participant.

Romance, Weiss, and Bockovan (1986), in a study that did not differentiate types of youth sport experience, obtained limited evidence that sport participation is negatively correlated with fifth graders' moral reasoning maturity. The results, however, were inconsistent; a negative correlation was found between length of sport involvement and maturity of moral reasoning in response to hypothetical "sport" dilemmas but not to "life" dilemmas. In contrast, Horrocks (1979) found a positive correlation between children's sport involvement and maturity of reasoning about a hypothetical sport dilemma. Future research should include qualitative assessment of children's sport experience in light of such variables as sport structures and coaching styles, rather than simply employing a unidimensional index of participation.

**Moral reasoning and behavioral tendencies.** Do children with more mature moral reasoning act differently than those with less mature reasoning? This question also grew out of studies with older subjects where evidence exists that athletes with less mature moral reasoning are more likely to exhibit aggression on the basketball court than more mature athletes (Bredemeier & Shields, (1984b). Similarly, athletes with less mature reasoning view aggressive acts as more legitimate than their more mature counterparts (Bredemeier, 1985).

Bredemeier (in press-a) investigated the relationship between children's moral reasoning and their tendencies to behave assertively, aggressively, and submissively, both in sport and in other life contexts. The sample population included 106 children in the fourth through seventh grade, drawn from the same summer sport camp referred to earlier. Results indicated that children's moral reasoning scores were predictive of self-reported assertive and aggressive action tendencies in both sport and daily life contexts. Children who were relatively mature in their moral reasoning described themselves as more assertive and less aggressive in response to conflict situations than did children with less mature reasoning.

In another study of sport camp participants, Bredemeier, Weiss, Shields, and Cooper (in press-a) showed 78 children slides of potentially injurious sport acts and asked the children questions designed to reveal their perceptions of legitimacy. Results paralleled those with college students: Children with less mature moral reasoning judged a significantly greater number of aggressive acts to be legitimate than their more mature peers. Although this study does not address action directly, it does so indirectly because children who perceive an act as legitimate are probably more likely to engage in it than children who judge it to be illegitimate.

**Moral education.** Current empirical research suggests that sport is an ambiguous context that may have a negative impact on moral development. If moral development is adopted as a specific goal, however, can children's physical activity experiences provide grist for moral growth? To answer this question, Bredemeier, Weiss, Shields, and Shewchuk (in press) conducted a field experiment designed to explore the effectiveness of a moral development program in a summer sport camp setting. Children aged 5 to 7 were matched and randomly assigned to one of three conditions: a control group, a social learning group, and a structural/developmental group. During the 6-week intervention program, each group was provided the same curriculum and the same weekly moral themes (fair play, sharing, verbal and physical aggression, and righting wrongs).

Instructors in the control group employed traditional physical education pedagogy, encouraging conformity to game- or teacher-prescribed rules. Children in the social-learning class received reinforcement for prosocial behavior that was also modeled by the instructor and peers. Structural/developmental group instructors were trained according to Haan's (1978) interactional model to facilitate children's peer-oriented moral dialogues in response to dilemmas that arose in class.

Pre- to posttest measures of moral reasoning (intentionality and distributive justice) revealed a significant advance in the reasoning maturity of children in the social-learning and structural/developmental groups; no change occurred for the control group. Although significant differences between groups were not found, the within-group results were encouraging and seemed to suggest that moral growth was stimulated by theoretically grounded instructional strategies.

Romance, Weiss, and Bockovan (1986) conducted an intervention study employing fifth-grade students divided into experimental and control groups. For the experimental group, researchers constructed specific game-related teaching strategies based on guidelines from Haan's model. The control group was not exposed to the experimental intervention but played the same games for the same length of time. Before and after an 8-week intervention, children responded to four moral dilemmas, two set within sport contexts and two in daily life situations. Between-group analyses indicated that the experimental groups gained significantly more than the control group, which demonstrated no pre-post reasoning gains. Additionally, within-group analyses revealed that the experimental group improved significantly in their reasoning about sport but not daily life, moral dilemmas.

In summary, only a few investigators have examined the relationship between children's moral development and sport activity. With more and more children participating in organized sport programs, our limited knowledge is unfortunate. Nonetheless, some general recommendations can be drawn from structural/developmental theory for constructing sport experiences that may contribute to children's moral growth.

## PROMOTING MORAL GROWTH

Haan's research suggests that for an experience to be effective in promoting moral growth it must be *interpersonal*, the participants must perceive their *interdependence*, and there must be opportunity for *dialogue* and *negotiation* (Shields, 1980). Play, games, and sport can provide a unique context where all three of these conditions can be met.

Sport experiences are inherently interpersonal. Even individual sport activities take place in an interpersonal context, for the full activity experience extends beyond the moment of competition or performance, encompassing such dimensions as coach-player interactions, dialogue among peers during practice sessions, self-dialogue, and dialogue about the sport experience at home and with friends. Obviously, informal games are also saliently interpersonal.

The interpersonal context of sport must be brought explicitly to participants' awareness, yet an overemphasis on such interpersonal issues as team cohesion can sometimes result in a de-emphasis on individual uniqueness and value. Uniformity brought about by adult authority or peer pressure must be balanced by opportunity for individuation. By prescribing an interpersonal experience, Haan, Aerts, and Cooper (1985) point to the need for mutual discovery among participants so that each individual's strengths and vulnerabilities can be known. Situations must be structured so that self-expression and interpersonal sharing can take place.

Interactive physical activities also provide a context for experiencing interdependency. Participants must cooperate and rely on each other. In informally structured settings, such as a pick-up game of basketball during recess, inter-dependency works as a good regulator of moral balance. Each team needs the other if the game is to continue; consequently, moral violations rarely become excessive. If one team seriously violates unspoken norms of play and thereby upsets the balance, the other team may terminate the game. In more formally structured settings, the interdependency between teams is emphasized less often, but correspondingly greater stress is placed on intrateam interdependency. Practice drills, for example, often highlight how one player's successful performance is dependent not only on his or her own skill but also on that of others whose actions must be coordinated. Though children's role-taking ability limits their capacity to perceive and coordinate role assignments (Coakley & Bredemeier, in press), the concept of interdependency is clear. The interdependent character of sport activity can be highlighted by providing "superordinate" goals (Sherif & Sherif, 1953) that cannot be obtained unless everyone contributes in some way.

In addition to being interpersonal and interdependent, those experiences that are likely to foster moral growth will be punctuated with dialogue and negotiation. Unfortunately, it is precisely this dialogical dynamic that is progressively re-moved as one shifts from games to sports and from less competitive, informal sport to more elite, structured sport. Moral discussions pertinent to such issues as what should be done about rule violations, when and why participants should risk injury, who should play, and on what basis rewards should be distributed are rare, even among those involved with children's programs.

Limited opportunities for moral dialogue can be expanded by affirming the quality of the activity experience over the importance of performance outcome. Typically, rich possibilities for moral dialogue and negotiation are consumed by instrumental concerns, and discussion is focused narrowly on such task-oriented topics as routine announcements, skill development, and play strategy. Moral growth can be significantly influenced by a youth sport structure that facilitates moral dialogue and negotiation oriented toward the interpersonal, interdependent processes of participation.

## REFERENCES

Alston, W. (1971). Comments on Kohlberg's "From is to ought." In T. Mischel (Ed.), *Cognitive development and epistemology* (pp. 269–284). New York: Academic Press.

Aron, I. (1977). Moral philosophy and moral education: A critique of Kohlberg's theory. *School Review, 85*, 197–217.

Blanchard, B. (1946). A comparative analysis of secondary school boys' and girls' character and personality traits in physical education classes. *Research Quarterly, 47*, 33–39.

Blasi, A. (1980). Bridging moral cognition and moral action: A critical review of the literature. *Psychological Bulletin,* **88**, 1–45.

Bredemeier, B.J. (1985). Moral reasoning and the perceived legitimacy of intentionally injurious sport acts. *Journal of Sport Psychology,* **7**, 110–124.

Bredemeier, B.J. (in press-a). *Children's moral reasoning and their assertive, aggressive and submissive tendencies in sport and daily life.* Manuscript submitted for publication.

Bredemeier, B.J. (in press-b). *Divergence in children's moral reasoning about issues in daily life and sport specific contexts.* Manuscript submitted for publication.

Bredemeier, B.J., & Shields, D. (1983). *Body and balance: Developing moral structures through physical education.* Eugene, OR: Microform Publications, University of Oregon.

Bredemeier, B.J., & Shields, D. (1984a). Divergence in moral reasoning about sport and everyday life. *Sociology of Sport Journal,* **1**, 384–357.

Bredemeier, B.J., & Shields, D. (1984b). The utility of moral stage analysis in the understanding of athletic aggression. *Sociology of Sport Journal,* **1**, 138–149.

Bredemeier, B.J., & Shields, D.L. (1986a). Game reasoning and interactional morality. *Journal of Genetic Psychology,* **147**, 257–275.

Bredemeier, B.J., & Shields, D. (1986b). Moral growth among athletes and nonathletes: A comparison analysis. *Journal of Genetic Psychology,* **147**, 7–18.

Bredemeier, B.J., Weiss, M.R., Shields, D.L., & Cooper, B. (in press-a). *The relationship between children's legitimacy judgments and their moral reasoning, aggression tendencies and sport involvement.* Manuscript submitted for publication.

Bredemeier, B.J., Weiss, M.R., Shields, D.L., & Cooper, B. (in-press-b). *Sport involvement and children's moral reasoning and aggression tendencies.* Manuscript submitted for publication.

Bredemeier, B.J., Weiss, M.R., Shields, D.L., & Shewchuk, R.M. (in press). Promoting moral growth in a summer sport camp. *Journal of Moral Education.*

Coakley, J., & Bredemeier, B.J. (in press). Youth sports: Development of ethical practices. In J. Thomas & J. Nelson (Eds.), *Ethical practices in competitive sports.* Champaign, IL: Human Kinetics.

Figley, G. (1984). Moral education through physical education. *Quest,* **36**, 89–101.

Giebink, M.P., & McKenzie, T.L. (1985). Teaching sportsmanship in physical education and recreation: An analysis of intervention and generalization effects. *Journal of Teaching in Physical Education, 4,* 167–177.

Gilligan, C. (1982). *In a different voice: Psychological theory and women's development.* Cambridge, MA: Harvard University Press.

Haan, N. (1977). *A manual for interactional morality.* Unpublished manuscript, University of California, Berkeley.

Haan, N. (1978). Two moralities in action contexts: Relationship to thought, ego regulation, and development. *Journal of Personality and Social Psychology, 36,* 286–305.

Haan, N., Aerts, E., & Cooper, B. (1985). *On moral grounds.* New York: New York University Press.

Hall, E. (1981). *Moral development of athletes in sport specific and general social situations.* Unpublished doctoral dissertation, Texas Women's University, Denton.

Hartshorne, H., & May, M. (1928). *Studies in the nature of character: Vol. 1. Studies in deceit.* New York: Macmillan.

Hartshorne, H., May, M., & Maller, J. (1929). *Studies in the nature of character: Vol. 2. Studies in self-control.* New York: Macmillan.

Hartshorne, H., May, M., & Shuttleworth, F.K. (1930). *Studies in the nature of character: Vol. 3. Studies in the organization of character.* New York: Macmillan.

Horrocks, R. (1979). *The relationship of selected prosocial play behaviors in children to moral reasoning, youth sports participation, and perception of sportsmanship.* Unpublished doctoral dissertation, University of North Carolina, Greensboro.

Kleiber, D.A., & Roberts, G.C. (1981). The effects of sport experience in the development of social character: An exploratory investigation. *Journal of Sport Psychology, 3,* 114–122.

Kohlberg, L. (1976). Moral stages and moralization: The cognitive-developmental approach. In T. Lickona (Ed.), *Moral development and behavior: Theory, research and social issues* (pp. 31–53). New York: Holt, Rinehart and Winston.

Kohlberg, L. (1981). *Essays on moral development: Vol. 1. The philosophy of moral development.* San Francisco: Harper & Row.

Kohlberg, L. (1984). *Essays on moral development: Vol. 2. The psychology of moral development.* San Francisco: Harper & Row.

Loy, J.W. (1975). *The professionalization of attitudes toward play as a function of selected social identities and level of sport participation*. Paper presented at the international seminar on Play in Physical Education and Sport, Tel Aviv.

Maloney, T.L., & Petrie, B.M. (1974). Professionalization of attitudes toward play among Canadian school pupils as a function of sex, grade and athletic participation. *Journal of Leisure Research, 4*, 184–195.

Mantel, R.C., & Velden, V.L. (1974). The relationship between the professionalization of attitude toward play of preadolescent boys and participation in organized sport. In G.H. Sage (Ed.), *Sport and American society* (2nd ed.) (pp. 172–178). Reading, MA: Addison-Wesley.

McCloy, C.H. (1930). Character building through physical education. *Research Quarterly, 1*, 41–59.

Munsey, B. (1980). Cognitive-developmental theory of moral development: Metaethical issues. In B. Munsey (Ed.), *Moral development, moral education, and Kohlberg* (pp. 161–181). Birmingham, AL: Religious Education Press.

Orlick, T. (1981). Positive socialization via cooperative games. *Developmental Psychology, 17*, 426–429.

Petrie, B.M. (1971). Achievement orientation in adolescent attitudes toward play. *International Review of Sport Sociology, 6*, 89–99.

Piaget, J. (1932). *The moral judgment of the child*. New York: Harcourt and Brace.

Romance, T., Weiss, M., & Bockovan, J. (1986). A program to promote moral development through elementary school physical education. *Journal of Teachers of Physical Education, 5*(2), 126–136.

Sage, G.H. (1980). Orientations toward sport of male and female intercollegiate athletes. *Journal of Sport Psychology, 2*, 355–362.

Sherif, M., & Sherif, C. (1953). *Groups in harmony and tension*. New York: Harper & Row.

Shields, D. (1980). Education for moral action. *Religious Education, 75*, 129–142.

Shields, D. (1986). *Growing beyond prejudices*. Mystic, CT: Twenty-Third Publications.

Shweder, R. (1982). Review of Lawrence Kohlberg's "Essays on moral development: Vol. 1. The philosophy of moral development." *Contemporary Psychology, 27*, 421–424.

Simpson, E. (1974). Moral development research: A case study of scientific cultural bias. *Human Development, 17*, 81–106.

Simpson, E. (1983). Emile's moral development. *Human Development, 26,* 198–212.

Sullivan, E. (1977). A study of Kohlberg's structural theory of moral development: A critique of liberal social science ideology. *Human Development, 20,* 352–376.

Turiel, E. (1983). *The development of social knowledge: Morality and convention.* Cambridge, England: Cambridge University Press.

Webb, H. (1969). Professionalization of attitudes toward play among adolescents. In G.S. Kenyon (Ed.), *Aspects of contemporary sport sociology* (pp. 161–168). Chicago: The Athletic Institute.

# 8

# Developmental Perspectives of Motor Skill Performance in Children

Beverly D. Ulrich

Viewing children's performance of motor skills in perspective implies focusing on the interrelated elements that comprise the whole. The importance of such an approach suggests that anyone who interacts with children—whether researcher, practitioner, or parent—must understand that behavior observed (the whole) is a function of a variety of influences (the interrelated elements). Attempts to affect behavior must be shaped by knowing what these elements are as well as understanding that in a given performance situation each child's status on these elements is unique.

This chapter initially describes the observed changes in gross motor skills of children between the ages of 2-1/2 and 10. Subsequently, the influences of anatomical changes and environmental constraints on the acquisition and utilization of motor skills are addressed.

## SKILL DEVELOPMENT VIEWED AS A HIERARCHY

Normal development of one's repertoire of motor skills may be viewed as a hierarchy (see Figure 1). The neonatal period and infancy are characterized by the orderly appearance and subsequent disappearance of numerous reflexes. Performance of these reflexive movements, theoretically at least, form the neurological substrates upon which later movement patterns are based (Knott & Voss, 1968; Milani-Comparetti & Gidoni, 1967).

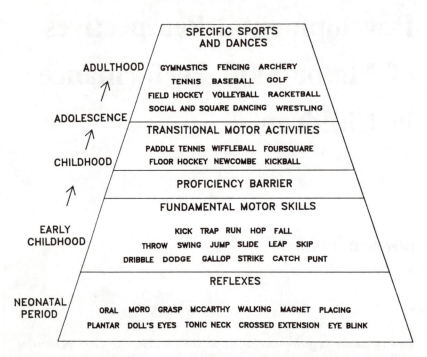

**Figure 1.** Sequential acquisition of motor skills. *Note.* Adapted from Seefeldt, 1980, p. 317.

During the early childhood years competence in performing motor skills such as throwing, catching, kicking, jumping, hopping, galloping, and skipping begins to develop. Such skills are referred to as fundamental motor skills because they form the foundation upon which all subsequent motor skills are based. By age 6, most children are proficient enough in these skills that they may be modified into transitional skills and used in the traditional games of childhood. Williams (1983) stated that most skills used in games, sports, and dances are actually combinations and modifications of these fundamental skills. For example, a lay-up in basketball may be conceptualized as a combination with modifications of a leap, hop, and overarm throw.

Transitional skills may be defined as simple combinations and variations of fundamental motor skills. They are used to play the traditional games of childhood and less complicated versions of specific sports. Games such as beach ball volleyball and one-bounce volleyball are simplified versions of the official sport of volleyball. They require the performer to execute a sport skill such as the forearm pass but with a larger, softer, and slower moving ball. Such skills are taught to and performed by children prior to their acquisition of sport-specific skills.

The transition from acquiring fundamental motor skills to performing variations of them and applying them in increasingly complex situations is not smooth for all children and is clearly not automatic. Children's progress depends on their learning experiences in combination with their biological development. Those who are not provided with the proper environment and opportunities to practice motor skills may encounter a proficiency barrier (Seefeldt, 1980). Participating in and learning more complex skills become extremely difficult if fundamental skills are poorly developed.

During late childhood most children learn sport-specific motor skills. The forearm pass in volleyball that the younger child performed after the ball bounced must now conform to universally accepted rules and be executed before the ball bounces. Skills such as the spike, block, and dig may be added to the child's volleyball skills repertoire.

## EARLY CHILDHOOD SKILL DEVELOPMENT

Rudimentary skill patterns that emerge during the early childhood years (ages 2-1/2 to 5-1/2) undergo progressive qualitative changes that lead to mature and more efficient movement patterns. These changes are sequential, orderly, and similar for most individuals and are referred to as intraskill sequences. Thus, researchers have begun to identify developmental sequences that characterize the acquisition of fundamental motor skills.

Current attempts to describe sequences in the development of basic motor skills emanate primarily from two universities and comprise two distinct approaches. Researchers at Michigan State University (Haubenstricker, Branta, & Seefeldt, 1983; Seefeldt & Haubenstricker, 1982) have taken the traditional method in which the actions of the total body are described. This approach implies that as change occurs, the interrelationships among body segments are sufficiently cohesive as to be characterized as a totality. In contrast, investigators at the University of Wisconsin (Halverson, 1983; Roberton, 1983; Williams, 1980) have utilized a component approach in which separate developmental sequences are determined for each relevant body segment, such as the forearm, arm, trunk, and leg. They contend that changes in the movement patterns of different body segments do not necessarily occur simultaneously and should therefore be analyzed separately.

Table 1 describes how the young child might look when initially able to perform the hop, as described via the total-body and component approaches. Similarities in the descriptions may be observed. For example, the arms are described in each as being held high and to the side of the body. A difference is apparent in that the component description more explicitly defines the movement of the support leg. Regardless of their differences, these researchers have clearly demonstrated the complex nature of change in the performance of fundamental motor skills.

One premise underlying descriptions of change in motor skills is that each higher stage or level results in a biomechanically more efficient performance. Recently support for this contention has been obtained via studies in which the product of performance was compared to the process or pattern of movement. Roberton, Halverson, and Erbaugh (1980) reported that the level of performance on four components of the overarm throw could be used in a regression

## Table 1

### Two Approaches to Describing Movement of the Body Segments During a Child's Earliest Successful Attempts to Perform a Hop

#### Total body approach[a]

Stage 1.  The nonsupport knee is flexed at 90° or less with the nonsupport thigh parallel to the surface. This position places the nonsupport foot in front of the body so that it may be used for support in the event that balance is lost. The body is held in an upright position with the arms flexed at the elbows. The hands are held near shoulder height and slightly to the side in a stabilizing position. Force production is generally limited so that little height or distance is achieved in a single hop.

#### Component approach[bc]

Arms component:

Step 1—*Bilateral inactive.* The arms are held bilaterally, usually high and out to the side, although other positions behind or in front of the body may occur. Any arm action is usually slight and not consistent.

Legs component:

Step 1—*Momentary flight.* The support knee and hip quickly flex, pulling (instead of projecting) the foot from the floor. The flight is momentary. Only one or two hops can be achieved. The swing leg is lifted high and held in an inactive position to the side or in front of the body.

[a]Haubenstricker, Henn, and Seefeldt, 1975.
[b]Halverson and Williams (cited in Roberton & Halverson, 1984).
[c]To date, sequences for the arms and legs only have been reported.

equation to account for 75% of the variance in throwing velocities for kindergarten boys and girls.

Continuing this line of investigation, others have demonstrated that the ability of movement form to account for quantitative performance may be influenced by the precision of the measurements used and the age of the performers. When the total-body approach (a more global measure) was used, the movement patterns of 2-1/2- to 5-year-olds accounted for a smaller, though still significant, proportion of the variance in their quantitative performance of the run and jump (Fountain, Ulrich, Haubenstricker, & Seefeldt, 1981; Haubenstricker, Branta, Ulrich, Brakora, & E-Lotfalian, 1984).

The developmental-sequence approach to describing the gross motor behavior of young children has become firmly established in academia and in practice. Research, however, is needed to determine how best to use the sequences as instructional tools. Should each stage be taught, for example, or only the mature level? From a theoretical perspective, Roberton (1978) has justifiably suggested the need to test the adherence of motor skill stages to criteria classically attributed to developmental stages (e.g., universality, intrasitivity, and structural wholeness). At issue is not whether the term *stage* is justifiable but how robust these descriptions are. Departures from any of these criteria may indeed be more interesting and tell us more about the development of motor skills as it differs between individuals or from development in other domains than would adherence.

## CHILDHOOD SKILL DEVELOPMENT

### Refining Basic Skills

During the elementary school years (ages 6 to 10), boys and girls clearly are using basic motor skills and many variations of them in games and situations of increasing complexity. However, most investigators of skill development have continued to ask them to perform simple throwing and running tasks in closed environments.

One of the reasons for continued interest in basic skills is the fact that data from such investigations suggest that for many, performance is still improving both qualitatively and quantitatively. Recent evidence refutes the long-held concept that by age 6, fundamental motor skills are mature.

Of eight fundamental motor skills tested by researchers at Michigan State using the total body description of sequences, 60% of 6-year-old boys and girls were able to perform only two skills at the mature level (Seefeldt & Haubenstricker, 1982). The running patterns of most boys and girls were classified as mature, as were boys' overarm throwing and girls' skipping patterns. In contrast, most girls still stepped with the ipsilateral foot when throwing, and boys used exaggerated and stiff body movements when skipping. Boys as well as girls could catch with hands only but not move their body in relation to the pathway of a ball thrown to their right or left. Striking a plastic ball with a light baseball bat resulted in a transfer of weight onto the ipsilateral foot for most boys and girls rather than the more efficient contralateral step.

Ulrich (1985) assessed the extent to which children between the ages of 3 and 10 demonstrated four movement elements of a mature overarm throw: the wind-up, step with the contralateral foot, diagonal follow-through, and sequential trunk rotation and derotation. Not until age 10 were 60% of the children able to integrate all four elements in their movement pattern.

When the component approach was used, Halverson, Roberton, and Langendorfer (1982) demonstrated that by age 13, only 29% of the females but 82% of the males had reached the advanced level of humerus action in the overarm throw. An advanced level of forearm action was demonstrated by only 12% of females and 41% of males; trunk action was assessed at the advanced level for 46% of males and none of the females. Only a few males and no females had reached an advanced level of performance in all components.

An examination of quantitative performances of children on skills such as throwing, running, and jumping shows a relatively linear increase in performance as age increases. For example, kindergarten-, first-, and second-grade-level subjects broad jumped an average of 33, 40, and 44 inches and threw a tennis ball 34, 38, and 42 feet per second, respectively (Halverson et al., 1982; Milne, Seefeldt, & Reuschlein, 1976). The average run velocities of 6-, 7-, 8-, and 9-year-old children were 14.8, 15.0., 15.9, and 16.0 feet per second (Hardin & Garcia, 1982).

The ages identified with specific levels of performance, as measured qualitatively and quantitatively, vary. This results from differences in protocol, measurement criteria, and sample populations. Regardless of their differences, in total such research suggests that most children can continue to benefit from instruction and practice of basic motor skills throughout the childhood years.

## Modifying Basic Skills Into Sport Skills

The importance of gradually modifying basic motor skills and using them in a wide variety of situations is suggested by the emphasis given them in most textbooks of elementary physical education. A weakness in the motor development literature, however, is a dearth of research that has investigated this aspect of skill development. Only a few researchers have utilized test items that expand on the protocol of requesting a simple throw for velocity or kick for distance. When basic skills are modified, they may better represent the movements older children use in daily games and play activities.

When accuracy is the goal of the overarm throw and a grip-sized ball is used, the task becomes similar to pitching or throwing the ball to a teammate in baseball or softball. Several studies required children to stand a specified distance from a wall target and throw for accuracy (Keogh, 1965; Van Slooten,

1974). Although the target size, distance, and ball varied, the results suggest that children become more accurate across ages 6 through 10.

Two reported studies involved a task that combined throwing for accuracy and fielding as a task or skill that simulates movements defensive players perform in baseball or softball. Children were asked to throw a grip-sized ball at a wall target (retrieving/catching the rebound) as frequently as possible in a specified time period. As with most motor skills studied, quantitative performance scores improved linearly across Grades K through 5 (Latchaw, 1954; Ulrich, 1984).

Quantitative performances on a few basketball and soccer skills have also been reported. As with other skills, an age relationship to performance was demonstrated (Hanson, 1966; Johnson, 1962; Ulrich, 1984).

When children's performances on sport-related skill items are measured, the specific nature of such skills suggests a need to look closely at the learning experiences of the children being assessed. Involvement in programs that provide sport-specific skill instruction such as Little League Baseball or Biddy Basketball should logically create a skill difference between participants and nonparticipants. The results of a recent study described such a difference. Ulrich (1984) compared the performance of participants and nonparticipants in organized sport on four sport-related motor tasks: the soccer dribble, soccer throw-in, playground ball dribble, and softball repeated throw and catch. Children in Grades K through 4 who participated in organized sports performed significantly better than nonparticipants in all tasks.

Results of a purely descriptive study, as was the one just cited, do not answer the question, Were skill differences a result of the sport participation or other factors, such as learning the skills from neighborhood friends or parents, which subsequently generated an interest in participating in organized sports? French (1985) recently found that boys aged 8 to 11 who participated in one season of basketball did not significantly improve their basketball skills. Although her subjects likely could perform simple basketball skills better than boys of a similar age who had no basketball experience, her results suggest the need to (a) identify the range of situations that provide for learning of sport skills and (b) acknowledge that improvement in motor skill cannot be assumed to result from participation in all organized sport programs.

The only published account of a longitudinal investigation of the development of sport-specific skills involved ice hockey (Macnab, 1979). Boys who were involved in highly competitive ice hockey from ages 8 to 12 and boys who were involved in less competitive hockey from ages 10 to 12 were assessed on six skating and puck-handling skills at regular intervals. A plot of the performance scores by year produced typical learning curves in that early learning was rapid (approximately the first 2 years for each group) with less dramatic improvement in performance scores thereafter. The slope of the curve was greater for more complex tasks and was similar in shape for both groups.

Of special interest is the finding that by their third year of involvement, the less competitive group performed more poorly than the competitive group did in their third year even though they were 2 years older. The difference likely resulted from the experimental group receiving twice as much training. Another possibility, however, is that some sports have a sensitive period. Ice hockey, for example, may be learned more easily if instruction begins in middle versus late childhood.

Knowing that performance of the skills previously cited improves with age explains little about individual variations in performance. Some relevant questions to be asked include, Is a significant gender difference in performance to be expected during childhood? Is the best performer at age 6 likely to be the best at age 10? Do earlier maturing children perform motor skills better than their later maturing peers? How do variations in the environment, such as the implements used to perform a skill, affect the movement pattern? These issues and others will be addressed in the following sections.

## GENDER DIFFERENCES IN MOTOR SKILL PERFORMANCE IN CHILDHOOD

Gender differences in the performance of motor skills have been addressed directly or indirectly since the 1930s, but the issue remains unresolved. When performance scores on motor tasks are compared, results regarding the significance of gender differences vary from study to study. If the "eyeball" or tally technique is used to summarize the results of many studies, the advantage is generally afforded males, particularly for object projection skills such as throwing and striking. Females are sometimes credited with an advantage in rhythmical locomotor skills such as skipping, galloping, and hopping. Furthermore, differences appear to be less pronounced during early childhood and become greater during the childhood years, particularly for throwing.

When the results of many studies are integrated and tested for statistical significance, gender differences are found for most items. Meta analysis, a recent advancement in the treatment of data, allows one to combine the results of many studies and apply statistical procedures to determine overall effects and effect sizes. Clark and Ewing (1985) applied this technique to over 60 studies involving gender comparisons for children between the ages of 3 and 10. Results indicated that males outperformed females in all gross motor tasks except some nonlocomotor (balance) items. The differences were greatest for overarm throwing and kicking and were smallest for jumping, running, and catching.

The cause of gender differences is not clear. Anatomical differences and socialization factors are two proposed reasons. Biomechanically, males appear to have an advantage. During these years they are taller, have a greater proportion of muscle and less fat, and have longer arms and forearms than girls (Malina, 1975; Tanner, 1962). These differences, however, are small. At age 5 boys are about 1 pound heavier than girls and about 2 pounds heavier by age 9.5. The average difference in height is 1/2 to 3/4 inches; males' arms are 3 to 4 millimeters longer and forearms 6 millimeters longer than females' (Haubenstricker & Sapp, 1980). Such factors may be insignificant individually; in combination, a statistically significant advantage for males may result.

Learning may affect motor skill development more than size does. In our society males receive more reinforcement for sport participation, are more frequently involved in organized sports, and spend more time practicing motor tasks than females do (Branta, Painter, & Kiger, 1987; Coakley, 1987). In an interesting test of the power of experience in performance, Grimditch and Sockolov (cited in Wilmore, 1982) asked 200 males and females aged 3 to 20 to throw a softball for distance with their nondominant hand. Not until age 10 to 12 was a significant gender difference in performance found. Practice and learning experiences undoubtedly also influence the gender differences usually found in performance during childhood.

Although gender differences are statistically significant, it is important to note that in practical terms the differences during childhood are considered by most experts to be nonsignificant, and much overlap exists. Plotting quantitative performance scores across time for boys and girls produces curves that are similar for most tasks and close together. Figure 2 displays data from two studies in which males 3 to 10 years of age were found to be significantly faster

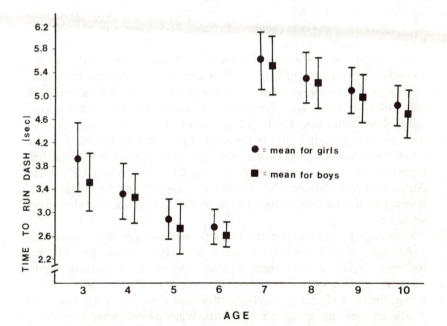

**Figure 2.**   Means plus and minus one standard deviation for boys and girls on the run for speed. Distance equals 30 feet for ages 3–6; 40 yards for ages 7–10. *Note.* Data from Branta, Haubenstricker, & Seefeldt, 1984; Morris, Williams, Atwater, & Wilmore, 1982.

runners than females of the same age. The considerable overlap in performance scores suggests that a large number of girls perform as well as or better than some boys. Conversely, many boys' skill levels are closer to the mean for girls than boys. For skill instruction or play situations, level of individual skill is more useful than gender for grouping.

## VARIABILITY IN PERFORMANCES

The concept of variability in performance is critical to understanding motor skill development. Mean scores, commonly presented in the literature, give the false impression that all children develop in a lock-step manner. Three types of performance variability will be addressed here: (a) maintenance of one's relative position in a group over time, (b) deviation of individual scores from the group mean, and (c) variations in the rate at which individuals acquire skills.

Maintenance of one's position in a group over time must be studied via a longitudinal investigation. Because such studies are time-consuming and expensive, relatively few have been conducted; and the skills studied are limited to the run, jump, and throw (Glassow & Kruse, 1960; Halverson et al., 1982; Keogh, 1969; Rarick & Smoll, 1967). Correlations between performances in adjacent years may be considered moderately stable. Values cluster around the high .70s to .80s, with girls generally more stable in performance than boys. However, significant decreases in stability occur as the number of years between assessments increases.

Correlations for interyear performances of the run, jump, and throw meet recognized criteria for stability ($r = .50$, Bloom, 1964) but stability and predictability are not synonymous. Even a moderate correlation of .70 accounts for only 49% of the variability in performance and makes predicting future performance almost impossible. Clarke (1967) demonstrated this when he reported on the status of boys participating in school sport programs in Medford, Oregon. Of all boys cited by their coaches as being outstanding players during their elementary or junior high school years, only 25% were stars at both levels. Forty-five percent were stars during elementary school but not junior high years, whereas 30% were deemed stars during junior high but not their elementary years.

Representing motor skill performances with mean values masks the great variability displayed by individuals within any group. If one looks more closely at the range of scores about the mean, children in any one age group may actually demonstrate skill levels more similar to the mean of an adjacent higher or lower group. Figure 2 illustrates significant overlap for run scores when only the middle 68% of each group is represented. When the full range of scores is considered, interindividual variability is more apparent. For example, in one group of grade schoolers the best performer on a running task among second graders exceeded the mean of fourth graders, whereas the poorest second grade performer was slower than most kindergarten subjects (Ulrich, 1984).

Studies that have addressed change in qualitative performance of motor skills suggest that children acquire movement skills at an extremely variable rate. The developmental sequences discussed earlier appear to be the same for most people but the rate at which they pass through them is not. For example, Roberton (1978) assessed three components of the overarm throw performance of the same children in kindergarten, first, and second grade. During this period of time, 6% demonstrated progressive change on all three components, 20% progressed in two components, 39% in one, and 35% showed no progress or some regression. When retested 5 years later, few of the boys and none of the girls had reached an advanced level of throwing in all three components (Halverson et al., 1982).

## ANATOMICAL/STRUCTURAL CHANGES

### Body Size and Composition

The fact that age is significantly related to improvements in the performance of motor skills appears to reflect, in part at least, an increase in body size (Peterson, Reuschlein, & Seefeldt, 1974; Espenschade, 1963). Childhood is a period of relatively uniform increases in height and weight with an average annual increase of 2 to 2-1/2 inches and 5 to 7 pounds (Haubenstricker & Sapp, 1980). Longer body segments and greater muscle mass provide for longer strides and greater force production, so that children run faster and jump and throw farther.

The logic and statistical significance that support a relationship between growth factors and motor performance must be tempered by the fact that the amount of variance in performance for which differences in body size and composition can account is low to moderate. Espenschade (1963) estimated that for boys ages 12 to 15, approximately 25% of the variance in performance on the run, jump, and throw could be accounted for by a combination of age, height, and weight. During the childhood years, when the variability in size among boys and girls of similar ages is less, the amount of variance that can be noted is also less (Rarick & Oyster, 1964; Seils, 1951).

The magnitude of the relationship between body structure and performance varies based on the motor task performed. One variable that generally demonstrates a significant relationship to performance is percent body fat. Tasks that involve propelling the body, such as running and jumping, tend to have a low negative correlation to body fat (Cureton, Boileau, & Lohman, 1975; Hensley, East, & Stillwell, 1982). Tasks that involve propelling an object, such as throwing, tend to have a positive relationship to body size (Ismail, Christian, &

Kessler, 1963). The resultant implication is that larger, heavier children are stronger, and strength helps one to throw faster and farther. Indeed, body size correlates more highly to performance on specific strength tasks than to motor skill performances. One may expect that as the motor skill tested becomes more complex and control of body movements becomes more critical to performance, the relationship to body size may become less important.

Maturity status or progress toward biological maturation, as represented by skeletal age, has frequently been examined for its relationship to motor performance. Generally, earlier maturing children tend to perform motor tasks better than do late maturers. However, this relationship appears to be most true at the extreme ends of the maturity continuum and is more often significant for children close to or in adolescence (Malina, 1982). In addition, maturity status, which is interrelated with height and weight, reveals that it adds little to predicting performance when these variables are considered (Howell, 1979; Rarick & Oyster, 1964).

The low correlations that have been attained in the studies just cited support the concept that an increase in skill is not an inevitable by-product of increased body size. Although growth variables seem to provide little predictive value, their statistical significance identifies them as contributors to the total set of factors that influence performance. Furthermore, one age group for which such variables may be particularly salient has received little attention.

Virtually no investigations have addressed the relationship between structural changes and the development of motor skills during early childhood. During these years, proportions of body fat decrease and bone and muscle increase. New skills emerge and patterns of movement change rapidly. The emergence of many of these skills traditionally has been attributed to increased strength and postural control. Recent theoretical attempts to apply systems principles to skill acquisition (Kugler, Kelso, & Turvey, 1982; Thelen, 1987) provide a basis for elaborating the possible subsystems that set the stage for skills to emerge and subsequently for testing them to see which are indeed rate-limiting and which are not.

## Scaling Equipment to the Size of the User

The relationship between a child's body size and motor performance has frequently been investigated. One very logical extension of that, the effect of the size of the equipment the child uses on performance of motor skills, has received little empirical attention. Physical educators and recreational personnel frequently adjust the equipment and/or rules based on their perceptions of a more proper fit to the size of the participants. Pedagogical experts suggest considering the size of one's students when purchasing equipment and provide modified rules for sport activities. Although such adaptations may be logical, few are based on research.

That children are smaller in absolute size and strength than adults is obvious, though what this means to performance may not be. In basketball, for example, the average male adult's height is approximately 58% of the height of a regulation basketball hoop. For the average male 9-year-old, that percentage is only 43. Essentially, the child must apply greater force to hit the same target as the adult because the ball must travel a greater distance. Several factors compound this absolute disadvantage. First, children have proportionately less muscle per kilogram of body weight than adults. Second, relative proportions of trunk and limb segments differ, which may change the length of resistance and force arms (Teeple, 1976). Ward and Groppel (1980) noted that success in learning and performing skills that utilize implements depends partly on the performer's ability to accelerate and decelerate the implement, that is, to demonstrate control. Biomechanically, children are at a great disadvantage when they must use equipment and rules designed for adults.

Recently, research has been conducted on modifying the size of the basketball for women, which may have parallel implications for modifying the ball for children. In 1978 a basketball that was 1 inch smaller in circumference and 2-1/2 ounces lighter than regulation was introduced by a sporting goods company. This "women's" ball was designed to increase control by providing proportionately greater hand contact with the ball and requiring less force for shooting, dribbling, and passing. In 1983 and 1984 several studies were conducted to determine the ability of this ball to meet the expectations set for it (Dailey & Harris, 1984; Husak, 1983). Results generally favored the smaller ball, which was found more frequently to improve passing and dribbling skills than shooting skills.

The significant effects found favoring a smaller ball for adolescent and adult females suggest that a smaller ball may also enhance children's performances. Children, being smaller, should gain similar control advantages. Most children also have accrued fewer years of experience with the larger ball, which was felt to be an interfering factor in studies with older players. A few investigations have addressed the issue of modifying basketball equipment for children, and some support has been found.

Haywood (1978) investigated the basketball passing and shooting performance of 9- to 12-year-old boys and girls when two different sized balls were used. Males and females at all ages scored better on the passing task when they used a junior basketball than when they used the regulation ball. Nine- and 10-year-old boys and girls performed better on the shooting task with the smaller ball, but 11- and 12-year-olds did better with the larger ball. Isaacs and Karpman (1981) assessed the ability of 8- and 9-year-old children to make a basket when the height was set at 8 and 10 feet. They found their subjects were five times as likely to make the shot when the basket was lower.

Results of the only experimental study involving modified basketball equipment for children suggest that children can improve their basketball shooting skills equally well with modified or regulation equipment (Stinar, 1982). Boys and girls in the fifth and sixth grades were assigned to either an experimental group that used a smaller basketball and 8-foot hoop or to a control group that used regulation equipment for 6 weeks of instruction. Both groups improved as a result of instruction but were not different from each other. From the studies involving children, modified basketball equipment appears to improve basketball skills. Also, modifications seem most beneficial for younger and probably less experienced performers.

To maximize skill performance, children of different skill levels and sizes may need different sized equipment; one size does not fit all. Wright (1967), for example, examined the effects of using lightweight and standard weight equipment on the acquisition of four sport skills for boys and girls. Results indicated that the younger (age 7) girls learned more by using the lighter equipment. Older (age 8) girls learned equally well with either weight equipment, but all boys learned more when standard equipment was used.

One of the most promising approaches to understanding how the size and weight of equipment can affect performance is by observing their effect on form or the pattern of movement. When modified equipment is used, a practical concern is the possibility of making the transition to regulation equipment difficult. However, if the modified equipment facilitates acquisition of proper form, this transition may be easier than breaking bad habits acquired by using implements that were too heavy or awkward to control. Halverson (1966) observed youngsters regress from relatively mature form in a sidearm strike with a light implement to a less efficient movement pattern with a heavier piece of equipment. Children who are forced to learn tennis with an adult-sized racket tend to adduct their striking arm and lean their trunk away from the ball when hitting, which is an inefficient movement pattern (Ward & Groppel, 1980).

A biomechanical analysis of the effects of varying the ball size and basket height on the shooting skill of seventh-grade boys is currently being conducted by an investigator at the University of North Carolina, Greensboro (Satern, February, 1986). The interrelationships of the body segments at various points in the free throw will be compared when regulation and modified equipment are used. The results of this study should provide a first step toward investigating the effects of equipment modifications on qualitative performance.

The effects of modifying sport equipment on children's acquisition of sport skills is a relatively unresearched area. Certainly children's immediate environments affect their performance. The attempts that have been made to document the effects of equipment modifications lend some support to the advantages of scaling equipment to the size of the user. However, not all modifications have been advantageous. Further study is clearly needed to provide an optimal environment in which children can acquire and utilize motor skills. The questions that need to be addressed include the following:

- What are the relative effects of modifying a piece of equipment, such as the ball in soccer, on *all* skills associated with the sport, such as dribbling, heading, and shooting?

- How do modifications affect the qualitative movement patterns of the user?

- When equipment is reduced in size to better fit the young child's smaller body size, how and when can the transition to regulation size equipment be made most effectively?

- When equipment can be modified to meet individual needs (e.g., the tennis racket), can formulas be developed that consider parameters such as hand diameter; arm, wrist, and shoulder strength; body mass; and body segment ratios?

## SUMMARY

Research suggests that changes in the qualitative and quantitative performance of motor skills of children are age-related. However, these changes are clearly not age-dependent. Increases in body size and changes in proportions provide a basis for acquiring and improving skills, but children's environments and learning experiences also affect their skill acquisition. Variability in performance among children is a rule, and individual skill assessments, rather than age or gender, provide a better means for classifying children for instruction or game play.

Some suggestions for research that extend previous work have been given throughout this chapter. The title and introduction, however, reflect the assumption that motor skill development in the child results from many interrelated variables. Motor developmentalists, like sport psychologists, sociologists, and others, have tended to examine only those interrelated variables commonly identified with their subdiscipline. We can describe how movement patterns tend to change with age but know little about the interaction of motivation levels or social facilitation effects. Future research should encourage greater interdisciplinary collaboration. Understanding the "whole" child may be facilitated when interrelated and interdisciplinary variables are embedded in the research paradigm rather than extracted from the review of parallel but isolated investigations.

## REFERENCES

Bloom, B. (1964). *Stability and change in human characteristics*. New York: Wiley.

Branta, C., Haubenstricker, J., & Seefeldt, V. (1984). Age changes in motor skills during childhood and adolescence. In J. Terjung (Ed.), *Exercise and sport sciences reviews* (Vol. 12, pp. 467–520). Lexington, MA: Collamore Press.

Branta, C., Painter, M., & Kiger, J. (1987). Gender differences in play patterns and sport participation of North American youth. In D. Gould & M.R. Weiss (Eds.), *Advances in pediatric sport sciences: Vol. 2. Behavioral issues* (pp. 25–42). Champaign, IL: Human Kinetics.

Clark, J., & Ewing, M. (1985, May). *A meta-analysis of gender differences and similarities in the gross motor skill performances of prepubescent children*. Paper presented at the annual meeting of the North American Society for the Psychology of Sport and Physical Activity, Gulf Park, MS.

Clarke, H. (1967). Characteristics of the young athlete: A longitudinal look. In *AMA Proceedings of the Eighth Annual Conference on the Medical Aspects of Sports—1966* (pp. 49–57). Chicago: American Medical Association.

Coakley, J.J. (1987). Children and the sport socialization process. In D. Gould & M.R. Weiss (Eds.), *Advances in pediatric sport sciences: Vol. 2. Behavioral issues* (pp. 43–60). Champaign, IL: Human Kinetics.

Cureton, K., Boileau, R., & Lohman, T. (1975). Relationship between body composition measures and AAHPER test performances in young boys. *Research Quarterly, 46,* 218–229.

Dailey, J., & Harris, B. (1984). *Use of a smaller and lighter than regulation basketball with female participants in Grades 7 through 12*. Unpublished manuscript, Bowling Green State University, Health and Physical Education Department, Bowling Green, OH.

Espenschade, A. (1963). Restudy of relationships between physical performances of school children and age, height, and weight. *Research Quarterly, 34,* 144–153.

Fountain, C., Ulrich, B., Haubenstricker, J., & Seefeldt, V. (1981, March). *Relationship of developmental stage and running velocity in children 2-1/2 to 5 years of age*. Paper presented at the annual convention of the Midwest District of the American Alliance for Health, Physical Education, Recreation, and Dance, Rosemont, IL.

French, K. (1985, April). *Motor performance development*. Paper presented at the annual conference of the American Alliance for Health, Physical Education, Recreation, and Dance, Atlanta, GA.

Glassow, R., & Kruse, P. (1960). Motor performance of girls age 6 to 14 years. *Research Quarterly, 31,* 426–433.

Halverson, L. (1966). Development of motor patterns in young children. *Quest, 6,* 44–53.

Halverson, L. (1983). *Observing children's motor development in action.* Eugene, OR: Microform Publications.

Halverson, L., Roberton, M.A., & Langendorfer, S. (1982). Development of the overarm throw: Movement and ball velocity changes by seventh grade. *Research Quarterly for Exercise and Sport,* **53**, 198–205.

Hanson, M. (1966). Motor performance testing of elementary school age children. *Dissertation Abstracts International,* **27**, 102A. (University Microfilms No. 66-05, 844)

Hardin, D., & Garcia, M. (1982). Diagnostic performance tests for elementary children—Grades 1 to 4. *Journal of Health, Physical Education, Recreation, and Dance,* **53**, 48–49.

Haubenstricker, J., Branta, C., & Seefeldt, V. (1983, May). *Preliminary validation of developmental sequences for throwing and catching.* Paper presented at the annual meeting of the North American Society for the Psychology of Sport and Physical Activity, East Lansing, MI.

Haubenstricker, J., Branta, C., Ulrich, B., Brakora, L., & E-Lotfalian, A. (1984, February). *Quantitative and qualitative analysis of jumping behavior in young children.* Paper presented at the annual convention of the Midwest District of the American Alliance for Health, Physical Education, Recreation, and Dance, Indianapolis, IN.

Haubenstricker, J., Henn, L., & Seefeldt, V. (1975). *Developmental stages of hopping.* Unpublished manuscript, Michigan State University, Department of Health and Physical Education, East Lansing.

Haubenstricker, J., & Sapp, M. (1980, April). *A longitudinal look at physical growth and motor performance: Implications for elementary and middle school activity programs.* Paper presented at the annual meeting of the American Alliance for Health, Physical Education, Recreation, and Dance, Detroit, MI.

Haywood, K. (1978). *Children's basketball performance with regulation and junior-sized basketballs* (Report No. Ed. 164 452). St. Louis, MO: University of Missouri, Physical Education Department.

Hensley, L., East, W., & Stillwell, J. (1982). Body fatness and motor performance during preadolescence. *Research Quarterly for Exercise and Sport,* **53**, 133–140.

Howell, R. (1979). *The relationship between motor performance, physical growth, and skeletal age in boys nine through twelve years of age.* Unpublished master's thesis, Michigan State University, East Lansing.

Husak, W. (1983). *Ball size effects on the competitive performance of women basketball players (Phases I, II, III, and IV).* Unpublished manuscripts, California State University, Motor Behavior Laboratory, Long Beach.

Isaacs, L., & Karpman, M. (1981). Factors affecting children's basketball shooting performance: A log-linear analysis. *Carnegie Research Papers,* pp. 29–32.

Ismail, A., Christian, J., & Kessler, W. (1963). Body composition relative to motor aptitude for preadolescent boys. *Research Quarterly, 34,* 463–470.

Johnson, R. (1962). Measurement of achievement in fundamental skills of elementary school children. *Research Quarterly, 33,* 94–104.

Keogh, J. (1965). *Motor performance of elementary school children.* Unpublished manuscript, University of California, Los Angeles.

Keogh, J. (1969). *Changes in performance during early school years* (Tech. Rep. No. 2-69). Los Angeles: University of California, Department of Physical Education.

Knott, M., & Voss, D. (1968). *Proprioceptive neuromuscular facilitation.* New York: Harper and Row.

Kugler, P., Kelso, J.A.S., & Turvey, M. (1982). On the control and coordination of naturally developing systems. In J.A.S. Kelso & J. Clark (Eds.), *The development of movement control and coordination* (pp. 1–78). New York: Wiley.

Latchaw, M. (1954). Measuring selected motor skills in fourth, fifth, and sixth grades. *Research Quarterly, 25,* 439–449.

Macnab, R. (1979). A longitudinal study of ice hockey in boys aged 8–12. *Canadian Journal of Applied Sports Sciences, 4,* 11–17.

Malina, R. (1975). *Growth and development: The first twenty years.* Minneapolis, MN: Burgess.

Malina, R. (1982). Physical growth and maturity characteristics of young athletes. In R. Magill, M. Ash, & F. Smoll (Eds.), *Children in sport* (pp. 73–96). Champaign, IL: Human Kinetics.

Milani-Comparetti, A., & Gidoni, E. (1967). Routine developmental examination in normal and retarded children. *Developmental Medicine and Child Neurology, 9,* 631–638.

Milne, C., Seefeldt, V., & Reuschlein, P. (1976). Relationship between grade, sex, race, and motor performance in young children. *Research Quarterly, 47,* 726–730.

Morris, A., Williams, J., Atwater, A., & Wilmore, J. (1982). Age and sex differences in motor performance of 3 through 6 year old children. *Research Quarterly for Exercise and Sport, 53,* 214–221.

Peterson, K., Reuschlein, P., & Seefeldt, V. (1974, April). *Factor analysis of motor performance for kindergarten, first, and second grade children:*

*A tentative solution*. Paper presented at the annual meeting of the American Association for Health, Physical Education, and Recreation, Anaheim, CA.

Rarick, G.L., & Smoll, F. (1967). Stability of growth in strength and motor performance from childhood to adolescence. *Human Biology, 39*, 295–306.

Rarick, G.L., & Oyster, N. (1964). Physical maturity, muscular strength, and motor performance of young school-age boys. *Research Quarterly, 35*, 523–531.

Roberton, M.A. (1978). Longitudinal evidence for developmental stages in the forceful overarm throw. *Journal of Human Movement Studies, 4*, 167–175.

Roberton, M.A. (1983). Changing motor patterns during childhood. In J.R. Thomas (Ed.), *Motor development during childhood and adolescence* (pp. 48–90). Minneapolis, MN: Burgess.

Roberton, M.A., & Halverson, L. (1984). *Developing children: Their changing movement*. Philadelphia: Lea & Febiger.

Roberton, M.A., Halverson, L., & Erbaugh, S. (1980, May). *Interrelationships between developmental levels and ball velocity in the overarm throws of kindergarten children*. Paper presented at the annual meeting of the North American Society for the Psychology of Sport and Physical Activity, Boulder, CO.

Satern, M. (1986, February). Personal communication.

Seefeldt, V. (1980). Developmental motor patterns: Implications for elementary school physical education. In C. Nadeau, W. Halliwell, K. Newell, & G. Roberts (Eds.), *Psychology of motor behavior and sport—1979* (pp. 314–323). Champaign, IL: Human Kinetics.

Seefeldt, V., & Haubenstricker, J. (1982). Patterns, phases, or stages: An analytical model for the study of developmental movement. In J.A.S. Kelso & J.E. Clark (Eds.), *The development of movement control and co-ordination* (pp. 309–318). New York: John Wiley.

Seils, L. (1951). The relationship between measures of physical growth and gross motor performance of primary-grade children. *Research Quarterly, 22*, 244–260.

Stinar, R. (1982). The effects of modified and regulation basketball equipment on the shooting ability of nine- to twelve-year-old children. *Dissertation Abstracts International, 42*, 3502A. (University Microfilms No. 82-02, 877)

Tanner, J. (1962). *Growth at adolescence*. Oxford, England: Blackwell Scientific.

Teeple, J. (1976). Review of research in growth and motor development with implications for elementary school programs. *Illinois Journal of Health, Physical Education, and Recreation, 2*, 4–7.

Thelen, E. (1987). Development of coordinated movement: Implications for early human movement. In H.T.A. Whiting & M.G. Wade (Eds.), *Motor skill acquisition*. Amsterdam: North Holland.

Ulrich, B. (1984). *The developmental relationship between perceived and actual competence in motor ability and the relationship of each to motivation to participate in sport and physical activity*. Unpublished doctoral dissertation, Michigan State University, East Lansing.

Ulrich, D. (1985). *Test of gross motor development*. Austin, TX: Pro-Ed Publishing.

Van Slooten, P. (1974). Performance of selected motor-coordination tasks by young boys and girls in six socio-economic groups. *Dissertation Abstracts International, 35*, 876A. (University Microfilms No. 74-17, 819)

Ward, T., & Groppel, J. (1980). Sport implement selection: Can it be based upon anthropometric indicators? *Motor Skills: Theory Into Practice, 2*, 103–110.

Williams, H. (1983). *Perceptual and motor development*. Englewood Cliffs, NJ: Prentice-Hall.

Williams, K. (1980). Developmental characteristics of a forward roll. *Research Quarterly for Exercise and Sport, 51*, 703–713.

Wilmore, J. (1982). The female athlete. In R. Magill, M. Ash, & F. Smoll (Eds.), *Children in sport* (pp. 106–117). Champaign, IL: Human Kinetics.

Wright, E. (1967). Effect of light and heavy equipment on acquisition of sports-type skills by young children. *Research Quarterly, 39*, 705–714.

# 9

# Memory Development and Children's Sport Skill Acquisition

**Jere Dee Gallagher**
**Shirl Hoffman**

As the accomplished ice skater glides along the ice in a free-skating program, his or her attention is tuned to the expressive features of the program and to the series of skills about to be performed (M.L. Olmo, personal communication, April 1985). Each anticipated movement is planned in relation to the prevailing body position; if the skater is not in the correct body position, the subsequent skill is modified appropriately.

The expert's flexible performance stands in sharp contrast to that of the novice. For the novice the immediate concern is the ongoing movement. The expressive features of the program and the skills required even a few seconds later must be ignored in order to execute the movements presently occupying the neuromotor system. Unlike the expert, the novice is unable to anticipate breakdowns in performance on the basis of present body position. Instead, each movement and component in the program represents something of a surprise; unlike the expert who modifies her responses according to the probabilities of future catastrophes, the novice engineers modifications on an ad hoc basis.

Descriptions such as these can be very deceptive. If ages must be attached to the performance, the expert would be judged to be older than the novice. Yet, the first description could refer to Tiffany Chin when, at age 15, she placed third in the world championships. Priscilla Hill was 10 years old when she passed her eighth test in school figures and free skating to qualify for national competition. Likewise, the novice description could easily pertain to anyone more than double the age of Tiffany or Priscilla.

Even though this description is of an expert child and novice adult, we typically confound age and experience and consider children as novices and adults as experts. Consider the fundamental skill of locomotion. The young child's attention must be focused completely on the information fed back from the eyes and various proprioceptors to avoid falling. An uneven surface or a change in elevation spells disaster for the infant because the information-processing channels are preoccupied with the skill of stepping and maintaining balance, leaving the child vulnerable to even the slightest alteration in environmental condition. Similarly, though having mastered the fundamental skill of walking, the young child who ventures onto an ice-covered sidewalk the first time is once again forced to attend to the information associated with each successive takeoff and landing. Rather than smooth, relaxed, confident movements, the responses are hurried, jerky, and tentative. The well-honed motor program associated with walking is not generalized to the novel environment of slick ice. The adult, on the other hand, is able to adjust the motor program without conscious attention to avoid falling.

Such simple examples underscore two fundamental features of skilled performance. First, the execution of human skills depends on more than the consistent replication of a series of movements; the efficient gathering and processing of environmental and proprioceptive information are equally important. Detection of nuances involved in movement and the environment lies at the heart of skilled performance (Gibson & Rader, 1979). Through highly developed processing systems, humans can achieve an astonishing degree of speed and coordination in such acts as playing a piano, swinging a baseball bat, or dribbling a basketball. Largely because of efficient information storage and retrieval, movers are able to anticipate the future course of serially organized movements or an open skill to achieve maximum flexibility in meeting the contingencies in the environment. Thus the performer is able to smooth out what might have been a halting and staggered response to an overwhelming amount of uncertainty.

Second, adult and child learners are both similar and different. From an observational standpoint, adults and children can demonstrate all the marks of unskilled performance, yet the etiology of performance improvement may be markedly different in each case. For adults equipped with a mature, fully functioning neuromotor system, the principal deterrent to expert performance is a lack of effective task-specific strategies for achieving the goal, a deficiency remediable by practice undertaken in optimal environments. The child faces a similar problem in that he or she lacks the necessary experience with the task to develop the requisite performance strategies. But the child may also lack the basic capacities for developing and refining these strategies, a deficiency remediable only through normal physical and psychological maturation. Additionally, the child does not use the same learning strategies as an adult for performance improvement. Thus, the difference between the adult novice and expert performer of a skill is largely one of experience with the task at hand, whereas the difference between adult and child learners can be traced to a complex interaction of developmental and experiential factors.

Before proceeding, two major delimitations deserve mentioning. First, from one developmental perspective, the human organism is in a constant state of development. In the early phase of the developmental continuum (into early adulthood), progressive improvements in the capacities of the motor system are evident, whereas in the latter three quarters of development, reversal in the form of a gradual decline can be detected. From another perspective, the study of "development" is limited to only the progressive expansion and refinement of motor capacities; the deterioration in psychological and biological processes evidenced in later years is relegated to a separate subfield, gerontology or aging. In this chapter, development carries the latter connotation, hence the focus is on infants and children and the differences between this population and adults.

Second, although researchers tend to treat the development and acquisition of skill, the effects of age and experience, as independent and isolable variables, in real life they are presented in complex and highly interactive contexts. Although chronology is considered the driving force behind "developmental changes" observed in advancing years, separating purely maturational effects from those of experience is impossible in any practical sense. Indeed, "normal development" depends a great deal on a healthy interchange with the environment and enrichment activities gained through experience that challenge the neuromotor system and stimulate its refinement. This complex interaction of experience and biological/psychological maturation is recognized as an inescapable feature of problems in human motor development.

Although physiological maturational differences are important factors in motor skill acquisition, the focus of this chapter is on how memory and knowledge differences affect motor skill acquisition. Much previous developmental research (for review, see Thomas, 1986) has failed to concentrate on the child's knowledge (experience) and how the application of that knowledge affects current sports performance. Knowledge base is developed through learning, and learning is affected by the memory strategies with which the individual approaches the task. This chapter will first focus on the importance of memory strategy use in developing the knowledge base and how that affects sport outcome. It will conclude more specifically by considering how information concerning sport performance is used to develop expertise.

## MEMORY STRATEGY USE IN MOTOR SKILL ACQUISITION

A major concern of developmental research is whether or not children acquire expertise similarly to adults, and once they gain expertise whether or not their performances are also similar. This section first investigates the importance of memory and knowledge base in sport skill performance and then the acquisition of knowledge base.

### Importance of Memory and Knowledge Base

Memory is critically important in motor skill learning. Learners must attend to the environment in order to decide on the correct action. Subsequently, as they perform the movement they must gather information about the success/ failure of the movement. Analysis of this information is used to modify the plan for subsequent performances.

For example, memory affects selection of information from the environment. It not only determines what the learner pays attention to and what interpretations are attached to observed events, it affects the planning and imitation of movements, including those directed toward motionless environmental targets as well as those requiring precise timing with continually changing external events. The learner's memory capacity enables him or her to build on past experience— previously learned subskills integrated with present task demands to solve problems of present concern. Memory also accommodates the storage of information important in the formulation of novel responses required when the learner faces an unfamiliar set of conditions (Schmidt, 1976). Memory also plays an important part in the evaluation of movement-produced feedback that attends the execution of a skill, and the accuracy of such evaluations are thought to be critical in motor skill acquisition.

Not only is memory important in learning motor skills, but once the skills have been automated it is also important in sport skill performance. Keele (1982) has argued that fast-action sport skills are not perceptual motor skills but cognitive skills dependent on memory or knowledge base. Reaction to the start of the movement is unimportant, whereas the ability to anticipate and predict becomes critically important. Keele suggests that the redundancy inherent in fast-action skills is stored in memory, and the skilled person has quick access to the knowledge structures that allow prediction and anticipation of events. Returning to the example of the ice skater, he or she could predict failures in subsequent skills by considering current body position and appropriately modifying the succeeding skill. Recall commentator Dick Button's surprise when a skater performed a double- instead of a triple-lutz jump. The question then is how the performer was able to rapidly adapt the performance. In order to predict future performance, one must rely on past performances under similar environmental constraints. Therefore, depth and breadth of experience are tantamount to skilled performance.

## General Adult/Child Memory Differences

In the development of expertise, generalizable memory strategies are important to remember important task-relevant information efficiently during and between practice sessions. How often have we worked with young children and they either ignore task-relevant information from the last trial or have forgotten what they did during the last session? Barclay and Newell (1980) have demonstrated in an experimental environment that young children choose to ignore knowledge of results and consequently do not perform as efficiently as older children and adults. On the other hand, Gallagher and Thomas (1980) have shown that the young child can use, when required, knowledge of results to perform a movement task like adults do.

For improvement in task performance, the individual determines that a skilled action is necessary and selectively attends to task-relevant cues in sensory store, filtering out all irrelevant information. Following perception, the individual selects an appropriate response based on knowledge of the factors likely to affect outcome (traits, task, and strategy variables). After selecting a response, the individual activates a motor program, taking into account contextual information including the nature of initial conditions, desired outcomes, estimates of impending changes, and environmental invariants.

All of these operations depend upon fully operative, efficient information-processing systems that focus on memory development (see Thomas, 1980). Information processing can be classified into three general stages: stimulus identification, response selection, and response programming (Schmidt, 1982). At the stimulus identification stage, sensory store and perception are involved. To date, the research on sensory store has not demonstrated substantial developmental differences in visual, auditory, or kinesthetic sensory store (for a review, see Thomas & Gallagher, 1986). Developmental differences have, however, been found in perception.

The use and interpretation of the information in sensory store are termed *perception*. Some researchers have suggested that a developmental shift occurs in the hierarchy of the dominant sensory systems, with intrasensory discrimination increasing (Thomas & Thomas, 1980) and intersensory integration improving (Williams, 1983).

The shift from a reliance on kinesthetic to visual information has been suggested (Williams, 1973). Williams (1973) has noted that the 4-year-old is quite dependent on tactile-kinesthetic (bodily) cues in performing motor acts and that the child cannot fully and effectively use specific visual cues to regulate behavior successfully. However, by 7 or 8 years visual information predominates. On the basis of such findings, she has suggested that sensory-perceptual development in the young child is characterized by a shift in reliance on tactile kinesthetic or somatosensory information to information from the visual system as a basis for regulating or modifying motor behavior. This transition to visual dominance represents a shift from the use of input from sensory systems with relatively crude information-processing capacities to the use of input from a much more refined sensory system (Williams, 1983).

Some scholars doubt Williams's conclusions (Jones, 1981). Jones argues that little evidence exists for the view that touch is dominant in early life. His review, however, focused on the tactile-kinesthetic mode for shape identification (Bryant & Raz, 1975; Goodnow, 1971) and not for use in movement control. Whether or not a developmental transition from tactual to visual dependence actually occurs awaits further research.

An improvement in intrasensory discrimination has been documented. With age, children are more accurate with positioning a limb (Williams, Temple, & Bateman, 1979; Winther & Thomas, 1981b), tactile point discrimination (Van Dyne, 1973), and anticipation timing (Thomas, Gallagher, & Purvis, 1981). Improved discrimination within a sensory system gives the individual higher quality information on which to make decisions for motor program selection, parameterization of the program, or detection and correction of errors.

An improvement in intersensory integration occurs at one of three levels (Williams, 1983): automatic integration of basic sensory information, cognitive integration of stimulus information, and application of concepts across different systems. Millar (1974) suggests that intersensory development is related to the development of better processing strategies, whereas Bryant (1968) has proposed that improvement results from intrasensory functioning. Certainly both appear important.

After perception of the information, the learner/performer must select an appropriate response or modify the previous response. Response selection/ modification is dependent on an efficient memory system. Response programming translates the motor program into muscle commands. This phase is neurophysiologically based and not discussed here (for a developmental review, see Williams, 1981).

## Adult/Child Differences in Memory Strategy Use

The findings of studies on sensory mode dominance are complicated by the interactive effects of memory strategy. Sorting the differences between perception and memory strategy often can be difficult. The importance of memory strategy use was pointed out in two recent studies (Gallagher, 1980; Gallagher & Fisher, 1983). Asked to recall simple linear movements of varying amplitudes, children performed simple movements as accurately as adults, but their performance was impaired when the complexity of the task increased. For example, when required merely to reproduce a single linear arm movement, 5-, 7-, and 11-year olds were as accurate as 19-year-olds. However, when the series was increased to three and five movements, the younger children's performance deteriorated rapidly relative to the adults' performance (Gallagher, 1980,

Experiment 2). Although such differences might be explained on the basis of developmental changes in the ability to process and store kinesthetic input, they are better explained on the basis of differences in memory strategy usage.

Memory strategy usage may involve any or all of the following operations: selective attention, labeling, rehearsal, and organization. Selective attention serves in the perceptual encoding (labeling) of task-appropriate cues and in the control process during rehearsal and organization. The developmental trend associated with this control process is from overexclusiveness to overinclusiveness to selective attention (Ross, 1976). Attention to limited cues, regardless of their relevance to the task, describes the child up to 5 to 6 years of age (overexclusiveness). The child is unaware of most environmental cues (incidental memory recall is low). Between the ages of 6 to 7 years to 11 to 12 years, the child attends to the entire display without taking into account the appropriateness of the cues for task performance (overinclusiveness). Thus, the child constantly is distracted by irrelevant information, and incidental memory recall is high. Gibson and Rader (1979) have suggested that this high rate of incidental learning in the younger child may be the result of a failure to understand the task clearly. At approximately 11 years of age, children exhibit a more balanced attention pattern, selectively focusing on task-appropriate cues and ignoring irrelevant information.

The basis of such transformation in attentional strategies seems more the result of experience than fixed maturational constraints. Stratton (1977) demonstrated that for a rhythmical timing task, young children can selectively attend to task-appropriate cues if forced to deal with the cues early in learning. From a practical view, Stratton (1978) suggested that teachers evaluate task requirements, environmental demands, and teacher input as a way of improving attentional strategies. During the performance of most motor skills, a wealth of task-irrelevant cues and environmental demands confronts the learner. Available data (Stratton, 1977) suggest that younger children are more likely to acquire strategies of selective attention when high levels of interference are imposed early in the learning situation in a way that forces the child to attend to those cues that are task appropriate. Presumably this provides children with the requisite discrimination training that enables them to sort out relevant from irrelevant information. However, the irrelevant information cannot be presented at a level that prevents learning of the primary task (Polkis & Gallagher, 1986).

One category of information available to the learner is visual feedback. In a synthesis of the role of vision in motor control in young children, Hay (1979, 1984) conducted several studies investigating the effects of visual feedback on reaching. Hay (1979) had shown that the extent of the visually corrected part of the movement was smallest for the 5-year-olds but greatest for the 7-year-olds. Subsequently, older children (7- and 9-year-olds) performed more poorly than the 5-year-olds (although their variability of performance was great).

The younger children ignored the visual information during the movement (indicative of the overexclusive child), whereas the older child attempted to incorporate the feedback during the movement and therefore performed poorly.

Labeling is one aspect of perception, and increasing the meaningfulness of the label improves memory performance. Winther and Thomas (1981a) investigated the developmental effects of labeling a kinesthetically presented movement; their results substantiated Chi's (1976) notion of a developmentally linked labeling strategy. Younger children's (5-year-olds) performance improved when they were forced to label a movement meaningfully. Adult performance was hindered when forced to use an irrelevant label. Weiss (1983) expanded this to a more ecologically valid paradigm to find that younger children (5-year-olds) benefited more from a model who gave verbal labels.

Organization and rehearsal are required to maintain information in memory and transfer it to a coherent knowledge base. Organization is a strategy for combining information in a meaningful way in order to reduce the load on the memory system. Rehearsal is the process of continually reinstating the organized information in memory either by cognitive-symbolic or motor reproduction techniques. In adults, learning is facilitated by rehearsal of information optimally organized at input.

Research to date suggests that children do not spontaneously employ optimal organization strategies in processing cognitive-verbal material (Chi, 1978). The implication is that memory performance might be improved through imposition or instruction in appropriate organizational-rehearsal strategies. Data from motor development studies suggest that young children may be taught to organize and rehearse movement-related information in a way that improves accuracy of reproduction of criterion movements.

For example, Gallagher and Thomas (1986) found that 5-year-olds were unable to improve accuracy of reproduction regardless of the strategy imposed on the degree of inherent organization in the movement information presented. Seven-year-olds, however, could use organizational strategies effectively when the movements were presented in a highly organized manner, but they could not transfer the organizational strategy to a new task. Eleven-year-olds were able to use organizational strategies to improve recall of organized input but not unorganized input, whereas 19-year-olds were able to restructure the information regardless of the degree of inherent organization in the original information. The results partially support a number of similar studies that have tested mentally retarded children (Reid, 1980; Schroeder, 1981) and corroborate findings from a recent study by Gallagher and Thomas (1984). In the latter study, 5- and 7-year-olds, given a series of eight movements to recall, chose to rehearse them on an instance-by-instance basis, whereas 11- and 19-year-olds grouped the movements for recall. When forced to group the movements in a manner spontaneously employed by adults, the 5- and 7-year-olds improved their performance.

The imposition of memory strategies was of greater importance to younger children than to older children and adults. The older children and adults spontaneously employed the strategies, whereas younger children did not. Even though the 5-year-olds were presented with highly organized movement cues (short to long movements), they failed to recall the movements in the same order, suggesting that they did not consider the organizational pattern. Forcing rehearsal, on the other hand, aided recall in the 5-year-olds. The 7-year-olds could use the inherent organizational cues and could profit from imposition of a mature rehearsal strategy. The 11- and 19-year-olds could use the inherent organization of information to recall eight movements. Those older children and adults who were permitted to select their own organizational strategy grouped movements according to similarity of amplitude, the optimal strategy imposed on experimental groups.

The importance of memory strategy development is to aid understanding of age differences in the knowledge base. A child's knowledge base has been said to be deficient in at least three ways (Brown, 1982): the amount of information it contains, the organization and internal coherence of that information, and the number of available routes by which the information can be retrieved (familiarity). An impoverished knowledge base can influence speed of encoding, labeling, recognition/perception, and ease of search and retrieval. This becomes a problem not only of adequate use and control of the routes available to the system, but also of accessing and using the resources available (Brown, 1982; Brown & Campione, 1980). This is what Keele (1982) considers knowledge structures and what permits quick action via prediction and anticipation of the environment.

## Knowledge Base

That knowledge base is globally deficient in young children does not mean that children cannot develop a rich knowledge base in a special area (expertise). Closely related to the development of a knowledge base is the development of automatic use of the memory strategies discussed earlier. Chi (1982) found that a 5-year-old used a regular retrieval order for four trials when remembering children in her class. Retrieval was managed using seat position and row, not the taxonomic categories normally used by adults (age, grade, and sex). Nevertheless, the strategy proved successful. This might suggest that although the organization of that information was different from the organizational strategy used by adults, the information was highly familiar and easily accessible for the younger child. Familiarity with the material to be remembered appears to be critical in shaping the way knowledge is organized and may be independent of the learner's age. For example, a 4-1/2-year-old was observed to demonstrate a sophisticated strategy when recalling dinosaurs with which he was familiar (Chi & Koeske, 1983). The child sorted on an abstract dimension that zoologists had found to be basic to classification of the dinosaurs, a strategy normally not evident until at least 9 years of age. For the less familiar dinosaurs, however, the child sorted along more primitive dimensions. Apparently, the impressive performance with familiar dinosaurs was due to the well-organized and highly enriched representation that the child had of the stimulus materials. This knowledge base, however, did not generalize to new information, even where the material (dinosaurs) was taxonomically equivalent to the more familiar materials. As Brown (1982) has suggested, the child, although perhaps an expert in one domain, is generally a "universal novice." Adults, on the other hand, know how to become experts in new domains; they are able to demonstrate transfer from a wide variety of past experiences.

These findings may have implications for sport skill development in children. The knowledge base is highly structured in most sport settings. In fact, a child's ability to anticipate possible outcomes and select appropriate responses, operations dependent upon a viable knowledge base, is a major source of improved performance during the sport season. From the standpoint of knowledge structure, improvement is a function of the acquisition of production systems, a series of "if-then" rules weighted according to their likelihood of occurrence (Chi & Glaser, 1980). For example, the volleyball player learns to follow the rule, "If the ball is served deep to my area, then I should retreat backward to keep the ball in front of me." For the child, these rules might be simplified. In developing the concept of self-space the child follows the rule, "If someone comes near me, then I must move to a space where no one else is." This total process is useful in reducing the load of processing the multiplex of variables that must be taken into account in game/play contexts, resulting in increased speed and quality of the learner's response. Of course, increased skill in executing movements is also important, but the relationship between sport knowledge base and sport performance has only recently received attention. French (1985) found experts displayed more shooting skill and basketball knowledge than novices, but their major discriminating trait was decision making during game performance. Interestingly, across the season the performers improved their decision making without improving skill execution.

## DEVELOPMENT OF EXPERTISE

A number of researchers have described the process of skill learning as goal-directed problem solving (Bruner, 1973). In Gentile's (1972) formulation, unless the learner perceives the skill as a problem to be solved and the movement as the sole means of solution, learning will not occur. Problem solving often requires the recombination of consistent responses. Adams (1984) recently has explained the learning of complex movement sequences as the processes of acquiring hierarchically related subskills in which wholes are constructed out of existing parts. The same point was made two decades ago by developmentalist

Harry Kay, who noted that adults rarely learn skills *ab initio*; rather, they are always faced with building on subskills learned at an earlier time (Kay, 1969). Thus, the availability of the components is crucial for learning complex movement sequences.

If knowledge structures truly lie at the foundation of skilled performance, it is reasonable to hypothesize as Chase and Ericsson have (1982) that expertise in the broad domain of human skill can be explained not only on the basis of knowledge structure but also superior organization. Experience thus serves the learner by enabling him or her to organize a diverse and rich knowledge base about the skill available in long-term memory. This effectively increases working memory capacity, providing substantial advantages for the learner when confronted by the demand of a novel task as well as a familiar skill. Viewed broadly, mastery of a motor skill bears a striking similarity to mastery of a wide range of problems in the cognitive arena.

With practice, learners move gradually from a cognitive, verbal-motor phase of learning in which they are preoccupied with the immediate demands of the task to the associative stage where subskills are primitively combined to achieve the skill goal (Fitts, 1965). Ultimately, practice leads to the automation stage in which the learner can be described as voluntarily initiating responses but executing them involuntarily (Merrill, 1972).

The automation stage characterizes the performance of experts. The attention requirements of the task are reduced by more efficient processing of input, allowing more time and capacity to respond to unplanned contingencies. Eberts and Schneider (1980) have summarized the benefits of automatic processing as follows: less resources are required, processing is faster, the task is less susceptible to distraction, performance is more accurate, and the internal structures associated with the movements become more economical and efficient.

The major point for teachers and coaches of children is to consider the method of presentation of information, albeit whether the strategies are maturationally determined or affected by learning. The data suggest that younger children do not spontaneously use optimal memory strategies. Chi (1978) has proposed that the adoption of memory strategies with increased age may result from a complex set of processes involving the acquisition and perfection of the strategies themselves, linked with the development of content knowledge to which the strategies are applied. Thus we suggest that initial familiarity with the skill will first allow development of content knowledge, during which the control processes of selective attention, labeling, and rehearsal are then applied.

Once a general knowledge base is acquired, organization can occur. Some initial data recently obtained by Polkis and Gallagher (1986) support this hypothesis. The older age groups' (11- and 19-year-olds) performance was more effective when they had been randomly presented the tasks early in learning. Subsequently, they could select the appropriate task and perform the movement more rapidly. On the other hand, giving the younger child (5- and 7-year-olds) several trials of the same task before switching tasks facilitated later performance. Applying this to sport skill development, the teacher/coach should be certain the child has mastered the skill (process) of throwing at a stationary object. Advancing to throwing at a moving target, the child should practice several trials throwing at an object that moves at the same speed before changing speed. This would aid integration of task demands and response specifications that produce the desired outcome. Subsequent presentation of movement speeds presented randomly would then aid rapid decision making.

The nuances associated with information processing are, for the most part, "observable" only by inference in highly controlled experimental settings. The most immediately apparent aspect of skilled performance is the rapidity and smoothness of movement; the performer seems to have plenty of time to accomplish the requirements of the task (Bartlett, 1932). Such observable characteristics are merely manifestations of an improved internal processing system. Two major factors important in sport skill acquisition are rapid decision making and attention switching.

**Rapid Decision Making**

In many motor skills, performers are required not only to move rapidly but also to respond quickly to external events. In such skills as batting a pitched ball or receiving a tennis serve, the ability to make quick decisions is critical. Chase and Ericsson (1982) have suggested that the encoding and retrieval operations associated with such decisions are speeded up by practice.

An initial factor aiding rapid decision making is the predictability of an event occurring that requires the need for the skilled performance. Predictability of an event affects decision making of adults and children differently. Children can use sequence information and seem to do so in the same manner as adults (Kerr, Blanchard, & Miller, 1980). However, children appear to be helped by expected events and/or hurt by unexpected events more than adults (Kerr, 1979; Kerr et al., 1980), with the difference between expected and unexpected events decreasing as age increases. Kerr et al.'s results also suggested that children's sensitivity to repeated events decreases as age increases. Even though unexpected repeated events were no more likely than expected or repeated events, reaction time for the repeated signals was faster than reaction time for nonrepeated ones. The magnitude of the difference decreased as age increased, with no difference at all for adults.

Rapid decision making is especially important when movements must be timed to an external event. Success in such skills depends upon the performer's knowledge of the relationship between the time for movement performance and the timing of the external event. Performance on these types of tasks, often called coincident anticipation tasks, shows a reduction of error with age (Dorfman, 1977; Dunham, 1977; Haywood, 1977; Thomas et al., 1981). A similarly consistent finding is less error with increased speed (Haywood, 1977; Wade,

1980; Wrisberg & Mead, 1981, 1983). These studies have not determined if poorer anticipation timing (AT) abilities of younger children are due to an inability to estimate the stimulus speed (receptor AT) or their movement speed (effector AT). Receptor AT refers to the situation in which the individual anticipates the arrival of some critical event by watching or listening to the relevant parts of the environment. Effector AT refers to predicting the duration of planned movement. By matching effector and receptor AT, the individual can judge when to initiate the movement.

Most studies of AT have minimized the role of effector AT by employing a movement of small amplitude (e.g., simple button push) and focusing on receptor AT (e.g., speed of the stimulus moving down a linear trackway). Timing error is explained almost solely on the basis of the subjects' inability to predict the time course of the moving target. Two studies have shed light on the role of effector AT. Thomas et al. (1981) attributed the poorer AT timing performance they observed in younger children to decreased effector AT. Because younger children's lateness in responding correlated highly with reaction time, younger children may have pushed the button coincident with the signal arriving at the end light. The younger children initiated the button push coincident with the signal arriving at the end light and consequently failed to estimate the necessary movement time (effector AT).

Hoffman, Imwald, and Koller (1983) have also discussed the relative contributions of effector and receptor AT in such tasks. They examined throwing performances of 6-, 8-, and 10-year-olds under four environmental conditions: subject motionless, target motionless (Type 1); subject motionless, target moving (Type 2); subject moving, target motionless (Type 3); and subject moving, target moving (Type 4). Among their findings was a well-defined pattern of "late hits," trials in which the target that moved from right to left was struck on the two right quadrants. These late hits apparently accounted for the differences observed between task types. For example, the consistently lower accuracy scores observed for the Type 2 than Type 3 tasks paralleled the finding of a greater percentage of late hits for Type 2 than Type 3 tasks. Considered in isolation, the data suggested that the increases in task complexity were due largely to the increased demands placed on subjects' receptor anticipation capacity.

However, data collected on selected timing trials where the amplitude of the response was reduced to a single button push suggested a much different interpretation. Required only to depress a button when the target (Type 2) or their bodies (Type 3) were aligned with a standard reference point, subjects tended to be early, not late, and were earliest on Type 2, the condition in which the greatest percentage of late hits were observed in the throwing trials. Taken together, the data suggested that the performance breakdown observed during throwing trials was not so much the result of subjects' error in timing the future location of the target (receptor anticipation) as it was error in estimating the time required for moving the arm through the throwing motion, matched to projectile travel (effector anticipation). In both the Thomas et al. and Hoffman et al. studies, the conclusions relative to effector anticipation mechanisms have been reached largely on a *de facto* basis. Future studies should manipulate these two independent sources of timing error in a more direct methodology.

## Attention Switching

Aiding rapid decision making is attention switching. This gives the individual a wider base of information to select the skill or determine time/force/space requirements.

Attention relates perception to action and to a person's needs and motives (Gibson & Rader, 1979). Increased attention is the increasing ability to find structure and order in what is perceived. Klein (1976) and Wickens (1980) have suggested that attention switching, systematically monitoring various sources of information, is one aspect of a skill that must be learned with practice. Knowing what to attend to and when to attend to it often dictates the difference between success and failure. Not only must skilled performers direct their attention efficiently to a multitude of external events, they also must strategically allocate attention to a vast array of task-relevant, stored information. In reviewing the literature on development of skill memory, Chase and Ericsson (1982) agree with Klein and Wickens in this regard and suggest that attended information is automatically bound to the current context. This provides for relatively fast and direct access to knowledge structures relevant to the task. It appears that skilled individuals are able to associate information to be remembered with the large knowledge base in the domain of their experience and are able to index that information for speedy retrieval. Additionally, practice in storing and retrieving the information facilitates the speed of the processes.

In sport performance the expert must be able to switch attention rapidly from the performance of the skill (movement) to the game context and back to the skill in order to determine the appropriate tactical strategy. Acquisition of a generalized motor program (automation) allows the player to switch attention from control of movements required in the skill to higher order structures. Practice (experience) is the principal means by which the player learns to aportion his or her attention from the movement to the larger context in which that movement is being performed, using the contextual information to modify the motor programs controlling the movement. For example, the basketball player acquires not only the general program for dribbling a ball but also for switching attention to opposing players using the information to modify the height, speed, and direction of the dribble. Returning to the example of general space, the young child initially is able to dodge children as they enter the child's pathway. Later the child is able to switch attention from their current path to the gym at large to determine new and different paths to travel.

To this point we have discussed differences between (a) experts and novices and (b) children and adults in acquiring and performing motor skills. The final section investigates the type of information necessary for motor skill performance for both the child and adult for open and closed motor skills.

## USE OF INFORMATION IN SKILLED
## LEARNING AND PERFORMANCE

Newell and Barclay (1982) have identified two factors a person learns and remembers about their actions: (a) the association between the movement and its consequences and (b) knowledge of variables or factors that affect outcome.

The first involves a basic knowledge that the situation demands skilled action. In order to know this, the performer must also know how the characteristics of the task can be manipulated to meet the known goal. As Gentile (1972) has noted, the learner must clearly understand the goal of the skill and must perceive the movement and its underlying plan as the sole means of solving the motor problem; that is, the person must know that a purposeful action is required.

Developmentally, a difference in planning exists. For verbal information (Apple et al., 1972) and movements (Kelso, Goodman, Stamm, & Hayes, 1979), the ability to construct a plan to remember skills appears between 7 and 11 years of age. However, use of a movement strategy and plan selection does not appear until later in development (Gallagher & Thomas, 1981; Winther & Thomas, 1981b).

Action knowledge also refers to the learner's awareness of the *context* in which the task is to be performed. This includes the environmental cues that define the parameters of the task demands. To a large degree, context determines the action needed to perform successfully. In Schmidt's schema theory, context cues are used by the recall schema to set specifications and modify the generalized motor program. In Gentile's (1972) formulation, contextual cues include the regulatory stimulus subset, spatial and temporal characteristics of the environment to which the learner's movements must conform in order to attain the skill goal.

The second major category of knowledge includes variables directly affecting skilled performance: person, task, and strategy variables. Person variables involve the learner's knowledge of his or her enduring physical characteristics and ongoing actions (monitoring of response as well as knowing when the task is completed). Task variables are those that affect the difficulty and complexity of the act. These are acquired by actual experience on the task and/or generalized knowledge from experience on a class of tasks with similar characteristics. The last variable, strategy, refers to a person's problem-solving approach. Two features are important here: appropriation of behavior patterns useful in acquiring a successful action, and the responses that, through feedback, allow for modifying behavior.

This latter feature seems to include knowledge of results (KR), which has been shown to be important in several studies (for a review, see Salmoni, Schmidt, & Walter, 1984). Learners are unquestionably able to use information regarding outcome, presented in a reasonably precise and comprehensible form, to engineer modifications in successive responses. However, experiments typically employ tasks in which the connection between KR and the nature of movement modification required is fairly straightforward. For example, in a linear slide task, KR (which informs a learner that his or her previous response was short) not surprisingly tends to bring about a response of smaller amplitude on trial $n + 1$. It is important to note that KR does not provide the learner with the details of the movement sequence in reaching the goal (Adams, 1984), and many skills entail a relationship between the technique of the skill (movements) and the outcome that is not nearly so evident. Thus our attempt to make direct applications from KR research that utilizes simple positioning tasks to gymnastic, golf, or other sport tasks is likely to overstate the case (as it presently stands) for KR.

The reluctance of researchers to study the problem is compounded by the fact that learning and performance of some skills appear to depend upon timely and accurate knowledge of movement or performance (KP). Form-specific skills such as diving and gymnastics come immediately to mind. Skills in which maximal application of force are required, or skills in which the biomechanical properties of an optimal performance can readily be specified, may also be facilitated by KP.

Gentile (1972) has suggested that during "the fixation stage," when learners of closed skills are trying to produce the effective movement consistently, knowledge of performance is critical. Presumably, where the same environmental conditions remain on the next trial of the closed skill, learners will be able to use the KP to make appropriate modifications in their response. In open skills, however, KP is likely to be useless given that the nature of open skills virtually assumes that trial $n + 2$ will require a different movement than $n + 1$. Thus, Gentile has suggested that knowledge about the result (KR) or even about the regulatory conditions that were effective during the movement is the appropriate context for open skill feedback. Gentile's hypothesis, when tested in an appropriate experimental design, has received only partial support (Cooper & Rothstein, 1981; Del Rey, 1971; Wallace & Hagler, 1979).

Notably, young children, lacking experience and knowledge in a skill, are likely to understand movement outcome relationships even less and may lack an appropriate frame of reference for evaluating their movements. In such cases, KP takes on even more importance. The ability of children to process descriptive information regarding their movements or to relate that information to the movements planned for the preceding trial remains untested. (The possibilities of such cognitive operations as determinants of the course of skill development have been demonstrated by Gentile and Nacson, 1976.) Also, little is known regarding the meaning children attach to common descriptors of movement, even such common terms as "not fast enough," "tuck your body tighter," or "grip the racket tighter." The effectiveness of knowledge of performance for children will depend ultimately on the experimenter/teacher's understanding of the child's lexicon of movement technology.

Both types of information seem to be important in both open and closed skills, depending on the stage of learning and the characteristics of the task. The more restricted the movement possibilities are in a series of trials due to morphological constraints or those imposed by rules governing execution of the skill, and the less intertrial variability (response) is required, the more likely it is that KP will facilitate learning. KR is a requisite for learning, and augmented KR will increase its importance in direct relation to its diminished availability as an intrinsic feature of the task. The principal difference between open and closed skills is the relative importance of prediction and rapid decision making. Both open and closed skills require selection of the appropriate response and appropriate parameterization of a generalized motor program. For example, in golf, a general striking program is selected, and the learner decides the force, time, and space parameters. Likewise, after selecting a general program for batting, the individual selects the appropriate force, time, and space parameters. In the latter case, however, rapid decision making and timing the onset of the response are additional variables of importance. In either case, KP may be important in early learning of the program, whereas KR is important in determining the association between the movement and its consequences.

During early learning it appears that the learner is developing "content knowledge," a generalized knowledge base upon which more specific procedural knowledge can be developed. This procedural knowledge may include the acquisition of production systems, if-then standards, regarding the connection between initial conditions, response specifications, and outcomes (Schmidt, 1976). Adams has suggested that the learner may have difficulty evaluating the mechanics of the movement during the early stages of learning—an apparently critical operation for the development of the production systems underlying a recall schema—because the learner lacks a reliable perceptual trace (Adams, 1984). Thus novice learners benefit from KP in the very early stages of skill learning when an adequate schema is lacking.

Additionally, for closed sports, with breaks in the sequence of the game, greater decision-making time is available, thus fewer adult/child differences are expected (Thomas, 1986). However, for open skills, with the action continuous, prediction, preplanning, and rapid decision making are important. For this type of sport, players, even though children, must learn strategies to monitor predicted changes and probable responses.

Thomas, French, and Humphries (1985) suggest that the knowledgeable player uses the environmental cues in two ways. First, selective attention to task-appropriate cues is weighted as to probable game actions. Bard and Fleury

(1976) have demonstrated that expert and novice basketball players attend to different visual cues. Experts perceived offensive and defensive players, whereas novices only viewed offensive players. Second, these cues are used in advanced decision making for determining appropriate responses for game strategy. These strategies are abstract concepts.

We propose that the same information is given the individual involved in learning open or closed skills and varies dependent upon the stage of learning. During early learning, KP is important, whereas during later learning KR is necessary.

## CONCLUSIONS

The fact that young children generally perform motor skills less efficiently than adults is well documented on both an intuitive and empirical research basis. Many people suggest that motor performance improvement is due to neuro-motor maturation in general (Williams, 1981), and anatomical, physiological, and biomechanical changes (Newell, 1984). This chapter has expanded adult/child differences by focusing not on physical maturational components to development but by accentuating learning and experience differences.

Development of expertise can be facilitated by the teacher/coach. During early sport learning, the child needs first to learn the isolated skill performed under a variety of contextual conditions. For both open and closed skills, KP is of great importance for development of the motor program. When varying the context, several trials of a specific context should be presented.

During later learning, children should try to develop rapid decision making and attention switching for open skills and should stress performance repeatability for closed skills. At this stage KR and KP are important for both skill categories. KR is used to select time/space/force characteristics, whereas KP is used to detect and correct movement errors. For open skills, the random presentation of context is used in order to develop rapid decision making and attention switching.

From a lack of experience, the novice adult and child alike do not demonstrate an organized depth and breadth of domain-related knowledge. This affects selection of response and speed, consequently compounding the adult/child performance differences. Children are further penalized by the fact that they do not spontaneously use control processes of selective attention, labeling, and rehearsal. With knowledge of adult/child differences in development of expertise, the teacher/coach can structure the learning environment to require use of these control processes.

## REFERENCES

Adams, J.A. (1984). Learning of movement sequences. *Psychological Bulletin*, **96**, 3–28.

Apple, L.F., Cooper, R.G., McCarrell, N., Sims-Knight, J., Yussen, S.R., & Flavell, J.H. (1972). The development of the distinction between perceiving and memorizing. *Child Development, 43*, 1365–1381.

Barclay, C., & Newell, K. (1980). Children's processing of information in motor skill acquisition. *Journal of Experimental Child Psychology, 30*, 98–108.

Bard, C., & Fleury, M. (1976). Analysis of visual search activity during sport problem situations. *Journal of Human Movement Studies, 3*, 214–222.

Bartlett, F.C. (1932). *Remembering: A study in experimental and social psychology*. Cambridge: Cambridge University Press.

Brown, A. (1982). Learning and development: The problems of compatibility, access, and induction. *Human Development, 25*, 89–115.

Brown, A.L., & Campione, J.C. (1980). Inducing flexible thinking: A problem of access. In M. Friedman, S.D. Das, & N. O'Connor (Eds.), *Intelligence and learning* (pp. 85–130). New York: Plenum Press.

Bruner, J.S. (1973). Organization of early skilled action. *Child Development, 44*, 1–11.

Bryant, P.E. (1968). Comments on the design of developmental studies of cross-modal matching and cross-modal transfer. *Cortex, 4*, 127–137.

Bryant, P.E., & Raz, I. (1975). Visual and tactual perception of shape by young children. *Developmental Psychology, 11*, 525–526.

Chase, W.G., & Ericsson, K.A. (1982). Skill and working memory. In J.R. Anderson (Ed.), *The psychology of learning and motivation* (Vol. 16, pp. 1–58). New York: Academic Press.

Chi, M.T.H. (1976). Short-term memory limitations in children: Capacity or processing deficits? *Memory and Cognition, 4*, 559–572.

Chi, M.T.H. (1978). Knowledge structures and memory development. In R. Sigler (Ed.), *Children's thinking: What develops?* (pp. 73–96). Hillsdale, NJ: Erlbaum.

Chi, M.T.H. (1982). Knowledge development and memory performance. In M. Friedman, J.P. Das, & N. O'Connor (Eds.), *Intelligence and learning* (pp. 221–230). New York: Plenum Press.

Chi, M.T.H., & Glaser, R. (1980). The measurement of expertise: Analysis of the development of knowledge and skill as a basis for assessing achievement. In E.L. Baker & E.S. Quellmaly (Eds.), *Educational testing and evaluation* (pp. 37–47). Beverly Hills, CA: Sage Publications.

Chi, M.T.H., & Koeske, R.D. (1983). Network representation of a child's dinosaur knowledge. *Developmental Psychology, 19*, 29–39.

Cooper, L.K., & Rothstein, A.L. (1981). Videotape replay and the learning of skills in open and closed environments. *Research Quarterly for Exercise and Sport, 52,* 191–199.

Del Rey, P. (1971). The effects of videotaped feedback on form, accuracy, and latency in open and closed environments. *Journal of Motor Behavior, 3,* 281–288.

Dorfman, P.W. (1977). Timing and anticipation: A developmental perspective. *Journal of Motor Behavior, 9,* 67–69.

Dunham, P. (1977). Age, sex, speed, and practice in coincidence-anticipation performance of children. *Perceptual and Motor Skills, 145,* 187–193.

Eberts, R., & Schneider, W. (1980). *The automatic and controlled processing of temporal and spatial patterns* (Rep. No. 8003). Arlington, VA: Office of Naval Research.

Fitts, P.M. (1965). Factors in complex skill training. In R. Glaser (Ed.), *Training research and education* (pp. 253–263). New York: Wiley & Sons.

French, K.E. (1985). *The relation of knowledge development to children's basketball performance.* Unpublished doctoral dissertation, Louisiana State University, Baton Rouge.

Gallagher, J.D. (1980). *Adult-child motor performance differences: A developmental perspective of control processing deficits.* Unpublished doctoral dissertation, Louisiana State University, Baton Rouge.

Gallagher, J.D., & Fisher, J. (1983, May). *Effects of grouping and recoding on memory for a movement series.* Paper presented at the conference of the North American Society for the Psychology of Sport and Physical Activity, East Lansing, MI.

Gallagher, J.D., & Thomas, J.R. (1980). Effects of varying post-KR intervals upon children's motor performance. *Journal of Motor Behavior, 12,* 41–56.

Gallagher, J.D., & Thomas, J.R. (1981, April). *Developmental effects in preselected and constrained movements.* Paper presented at the convention of the American Alliance for Health, Physical Education, Recreation, and Dance, Boston, MA.

Gallagher, J.D., & Thomas, J.R. (1984). Rehearsal strategy effects on developmental differences for recall of a movement series. *Research Quarterly for Exercise and Sport, 55,* 123–128.

Gallagher, J.D., & Thomas, J.R. (1986). Developmental effects of grouping and recoding on learning a movement series. *Research Quarterly for Exercise and Sport, 7,* 117–127.

Gentile, A.M. (1972). A working model of skill acquisition with application to teaching. *Quest, 17,* 3–23.

Gentile, A.M., & Nacson, J. (1976). Organizational processes in motor control. In J. Keogh & R.S. Hutton (Eds.), *Exercise and sport sciences review* (Vol. 4, pp. 1–33). Santa Barbara, CA: Journal Publishing Affiliates.

Gibson, E., & Rader, N. (1979). Attention: The perceiver as performer. In G.A. Hale & M. Lewis (Eds.), *Attention and cognitive development* (pp. 1–21). New York: Plenum Press.

Goodnow, J.J. (1971). Eye and hand: Differential memory and its effect on matching. *Neuropsychologia, 9*, 89–95.

Hay, L. (1979). Spatial-temporal analysis of movements in children: Motor programs versus feedback in the development of reading. *Journal of Motor Behavior, 11*, 189–200.

Hay, L. (1984). Discontinuity in the development of motor control in children. In W. Priny & A.F. Sanders (Eds.), *Cognition and motor process* (pp. 351–360). New York: Springer-Verlag.

Haywood, K.M. (1977). Relative effects of knowledge of results treatments on coincidence-anticipation performance. *Journal of Motor Behavior, 7*, 271–274.

Hoffman, S.J., Imwold, C.H., & Koller, J.A. (1983). Accuracy and prediction in throwing: A taxonomic analysis of children's performance. *Research Quarterly for Exercise and Sport, 54*, 33–40.

Jones, B. (1981). The developmental significance of cross-modal matching. In R.D. Walk & H.L. Pick (Eds.), *Intersensory perception and sensory integration* (pp. 109–135). New York: Plenum Press.

Kay, H. (1969). The development of motor skills from birth to adolescence. In E.A. Bilodeau (Ed.), *Principles of skill acquisition*. New York: Academic Press.

Keele, S.W. (1982). Component analyses and conceptions of skill. In J.A.S. Kelso (Ed.), *Human motor behavior: An introduction* (pp. 143–160). Hillsdale, NJ: Erlbaum.

Kelso, J.A.S., Goddman, D., Stamm, C.L., & Hayes, C. (1979). Movement coding and memory in retarded children. *American Journal of Mental Deficiency, 83*, 601–611.

Kerr, B. (1979). Sequential predictability effects on intiation time and movement time for adults and children. *Journal of Motor Behavior, 11*, 71–79.

Kerr, B., Blanchard, C., & Miller, K. (1980). Children's use of sequence information in partially predictable reaction time sequence. *Journal of Experimental Child Psychology, 29*, 529–549.

Klein, R. (1976). Attention and movement. In G.E. Stelmach (Ed.), *Motor control: Issues and trends* (pp. 143–174). New York: Academic Press.

Merrill, M.D. (1972). Psychomotor taxonomies, classification and instructional theory. In R.N. Singer (Ed.), *Psychomotor domain* (pp. 385–414). Philadelphia: Lea & Febiger.

Millar, S. (1974). Tactile short-term memory by blind and sighted children. *British Journal of Psychology, 65,* 253–263.

Newell, K.M. (1984). Physical constraints to development of motor skills. In J.R. Thomas (Ed.), *Motor development during childhood and adolescence* (pp. 105–120). Minneapolis, MN: Burgess.

Newell, K.M., & Barclay, C.R. (1982). Developing knowledge about action. In J.A.S. Kelso & J.E. Clark (Eds.), *The development of movement control and co-ordination* (pp. 175–212). New York: John Wiley & Sons.

Polkis, G.A., & Gallagher, J.D. (1986, April). *Effects of contextual interference on motor skill acquisition across age.* Paper presented at the convention of the American Alliance for Health, Physical Education, Recreation, and Dance, Cincinnati, OH.

Reid, G. (1980). The effects of memory strategy instruction in short-term motor memory of the mentally retarded. *Journal of Motor Behavior, 12,* 221–228.

Ross, A. (1976). *Psychological aspects of learning disabilities and reading disorders.* New York: McGraw-Hill.

Salmoni, A.W., Schmidt, R.A., & Walter, C.B. (1984). Knowledge of results and motor learning: A review and critical reappraisal. *Psychological Bulletin, 95,* 355–386.

Schroeder, R.K. (1981). *The effects of rehearsal on information processing efficiency of severely/profoundly retarded normal individuals.* Unpublished doctoral dissertation, Louisiana State University, Baton Rouge.

Schmidt, R.A. (1976). The schema as a solution to some persistent problems in motor learning theory. In G.E. Stelmach (Ed.), *Motor control: Issues and trends* (pp. 41–66). New York: Academic Press.

Schmidt, R.A. (1982). *Motor control and learning: A behavioral emphasis.* Champaign, IL: Human Kinetics.

Stratton, R. (1977). Selective attention in a multiple response reaction time task. *Perceptual and Motor Skills, 44,* 889–890.

Stratton, R.K. (1978). Information processing deficits in children's motor performance: Implications for instruction. *Motor Skills: Theory into Practice, 3,* 49–55.

Thomas, J.R. (1980). Acquisition of motor skills: Information processing differences between adults and children. *Research Quarterly for Exercise and Sport, 51,* 158–175.

Thomas, J.R. (1986, January). *As children get older, motor performance gets better: The question is why?* Paper presented at the Gatorade Symposium, Tempe, AZ.

Thomas, J.R., French, K., & Humphries, C. (1985). *Children's development of sport skill knowledge and sport performance.* Unpublished manuscript, Louisiana State University, Baton Rouge.

Thomas, J.R., & Gallagher, J.D. (1986). Memory development and motor skill acquisition. In V. Seefeldt (Ed.), *Contributions of physical activity to human well being* (pp. 125–139). Reston, VA: AAHPERD Publications.

Van Dyne, H.J. (1973). Foundations of tactical perception in three to seven year olds. *Journal of the Association of Perception, 8,* 1–9.

Wade, M.G. (1980). Coincidence anticipation of young normal and handicapped children. *Journal of Motor Behavior, 12,* 103–112.

Wallace, S.A., & Hagler, R.W. (1979). Knowledge of performance and the learning of a closed motor skill. *Research Quarterly, 50,* 265–271.

Weiss, M. (1983). Modeling and motor performance: A developmental perspective. *Research Quarterly for Exercise and Sport, 54,* 190–197.

Wickens, C.D. (1980). The structure of processing resources. In R. Nickerson (Ed.), *Attention and performance VII* (pp. 239–251). Hillsdale, NJ: Erlbaum.

Williams, H.G. (1973). Perceptual-motor development in young children. In C. Corbin (Ed.), *A textbook of motor development* (pp. 111–150). Dubuque, IA: W.C. Brown.

Williams, H.G. (1981). Neurophysiological correlates of motor development: A review for practitioners. *Monograph of Motor Development: Theory into Practice, 3,* 29–38.

Williams, H.G. (1983). *Perceptual and motor development.* Englewood Cliffs, NJ: Prentice-Hall.

Williams, H., Temple, J., & Bateman, J. (1979). A test battery to assess intrasensory and intersensory development of young children. *Perceptual and Motor Skills, 48,* 643–659.

Winther, K.T., & Thomas, J.R. (1981a). Developmental differences in children's labeling of movement. *Journal of Motor Behavior, 13,* 77–90.

Winther, K.T., & Thomas, J.R. (1981b, April). *Knowledge of movement response made: Effects of development.* Paper presented at the convention of the American Alliance for Health, Physical Education, Recreation, and Dance, Boston, MA.

Wrisberg, C.A., & Mead, B.J. (1981). Anticipation of coincidence in children. A test of schema theory. *Perceptual and Motor Skills, 52*, 599–606.

Wrisberg, C.A., & Mead, B.J. (1983). Developing coincident timing skill in children: A comparison of training methods. *Research Quarterly for Exercise and Sport, 54*, 67–74.

# 10

# Children's Development of Posture and Balance Control: Changes in Motor Coordination and Sensory Integration

Marjorie H. Woollacott
Bettina Debû
Anne Shumway-Cook

Motor development in children is a complex process, dependent on the acquisition and refinement of two different types of motor abilities. These two abilities can be broadly defined under the umbrellas of (a) voluntary motor control, including abilities such as eye-hand coordination; and (b) automatic postural adjustments such as postural responses to stance perturbation. Almost all of the research to date on motor development in children has focused on the development of voluntary motor skills. However, investigators must realize that the efficient execution of a voluntary movement relies on the concomitant activation of an appropriate postural set, which is fundamental to accurate movement execution (Belenkii, Gurfinkel, & Paltsev, 1967; Cordo & Nashner, 1982; Lee, 1980). A large number of studies on the execution of voluntary movements in animals has shown that postural and voluntary movements are controlled by the same structure (the motor and premotor areas of the cortex) (Gahery & Massion, 1981; Legallet & Gahery, 1980; Massion & Gahery, 1979). In fact, the absence of a postural set has been shown to be a symptom associated with certain types of human nervous system dysfunction (Horak, Esselman, Anderson, & Lynch, 1984; Traub, Rothwell, & Marsden, 1980). The development of the postural response system is therefore likely to strongly influence the development of voluntary motor control.

Two issues are critical to the understanding of normal motor development: (a) the development of the postural control system itself and (b) the manner in which the postural and voluntary control systems' development are interrelated. This chapter will address the first issue in detail and report preliminary findings related to the second. Studies will be reviewed that analyze the development of postural systems from infancy through adulthood, and the premise will be developed that postural control systems, like voluntary control systems, show a developmental gradient in the cephalocaudal direction as children develop, with postural neuromuscular responses appearing first in the neck, then trunk, and finally the legs. We shall also explore the contribution of three sensory systems to balance control the visual, somatosensory, and vestibular systems. We shall describe the involvement of these systems in balance control in young children, with a possible dominance of visual inputs in children first learning to stand. In children of 4 to 6 years of age we shall see the ability to attenuate postural responses adaptively to changing environmental conditions begin to emerge. However, we shall see that the ability to balance when there is incongruence among sensory inputs does not seem to mature until 7 to 10 years of age.

## EVIDENCE FOR FUNCTIONAL POSTURAL CONTROL MECHANISMS IN THE NEWBORN

The following section will explore the research literature related to the first appearance of postural adjustments in infants. We will attempt to determine the extent to which two different mechanisms contribute to the development of appropriate connections that allow relevant sensory inputs to elicit appropriately organized postural muscle responses: (a) genetic predetermination and/or (b) experience during a trial-and-error learning period.

Previous research by Bower (1972, 1974), Yonas (1981), and others on infants' behavioral responses to rapidly expanding optical patterns, though not directly exploring the mechanisms underlying postural control, may give us a key to understanding postural development if reinterpreted with postural issues in mind. The authors cited have classified a variety of behaviors as responses to "looming" objects, with *looming* being defined by Butterworth (1982) as "accelerated optical expansion of a determined portion of the visual field." Bower and his colleagues (Bower, 1974; Bower, Broughton, & Moore, 1970) describe part of the behavioral response as the head moving backward and the arms raising, and conclude that it is a defensive reaction designed to protect the infant from approaching objects. They report observing behavioral responses to looming objects in newborns 6 to 9 days old and in infants 2 weeks old. More recently, Yonas (1981) has suggested a different interpretation for these backward head movements. He has shown that infants have a strong tendency to track moving contours, and he concludes that visual tracking of upward moving contours causes backward head movement, and thus a loss of balance and a compensatory raising of the arms.

We have reviewed this research because these responses seem similar to those observed in sitting and standing infants presented with similar optical flow patterns that simulate body sway (Butterworth & Hicks, 1977; Lee & Aronson, 1974). Lee and Aronson's now classic experiments on visual stimulation's effects on balance control aimed to test the balance of infants 13 to 16 months of age. The infants stood on a stable floor inside a room whose walls and ceiling could move forward or backward as a unit. Movement of the room caused visual feedback consistent with that experienced during body sway. A compensation for this nonexistent sway followed, resulting in a fall, staggering, or sway in the direction of optical movement. Butterworth and Hicks (1977) showed that sway responses of the trunk to this inappropriate visual feedback were also present in infants who could sit but not stand. They concluded that experience standing was not required for the development of these postural responses to forward or backward optical flow patterns. The head movements to expanding optic flow patterns found by Bower and Yonas are possibly similar in origin to the trunk and leg responses of the older children who can sit or stand independently. This could indicate a gradual cephalocaudal development of postural responses as children develop. However, experiments testing neck muscle responses to true postural destabilization are needed to determine if actual postural control of neck muscles is present in the newborn child.

From the results of their experiments with the moving room, Lee and Aronson (1974) conclude that infants first learning to stand use visual clues in maintaining posture. They believe that these cues are more potent than mechanical proprioceptive information because the conflict created by the discrepancy between mechanical and visual cues was, in the majority of children, dominated by vision. However, these authors base their conclusions on experiments in which children were only given dynamic *visual* stimuli. No children were tested under conditions in which proprioceptive cues were given in isolation or in situations in which proprioceptive cues indicated body sway whereas visual cues did not. Until these additional experiments are performed, researchers cannot state conclusively that visual cues are dominant in the control of posture in the young child.

## THE DEVELOPMENT OF POSTURAL
## MUSCLE RESPONSE SYNERGIES

In an effort to determine (a) the time course of the development of postural muscle response synergies and (b) the relative weighting of visual, proprioceptive, and vestibular inputs during the development of balance control in children, researchers (Forssberg & Nashner, 1982; Shumway-Cook & Woollacott, 1985; Woollacott, Debû, & Mowatt, 1985) have more recently used a hydraulically activated platform capable of movements in the anterior or posterior direction to disturb the child's balance momentarily (see Figure 1). In two separate studies in our own laboratory, children in a variety of age groups (15 to 31 months, 4 to 6 years, and 7 to 10 years in the first study and 4 to 5 months, 8 to 14 months, 2 to 3 years, 4 to 6 years, and 7 to 10 years in the second study) were studied and their responses compared to those of adults (Shumway-Cook & Woollacott, 1985; Woollacott et al., 1985). The youngest children, who could not stand, were tested seated, either independently or in an infant seat. In the first set of experiments only leg muscle responses were recorded; in the second set of experiments the onset latencies and temporal organization of responses

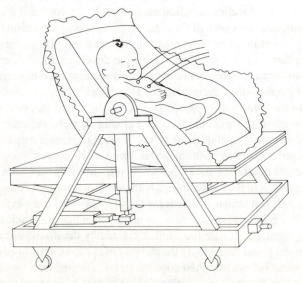

**Figure 1** Diagram of a child on the platform in an infant seat; the platform can move forward or backward in the horizontal plane. EMGs were recorded with surface electrodes.

of the leg, trunk, and neck muscles to platform movements were determined. Body sway was also measured using a belt at the hips that was attached to a potentiometer at the base of the platform via a rod. In addition, some of the trials were filmed in order to analyze joint angle changes biomechanically during the initial platform movement and subsequent compensatory muscle responses. In subsets of experiments, visual cues were removed (children wore opaque goggles), and in some cases the platform was made to rotate in exact proportion to body sway in the anterior or posterior direction (servoed condition). This kept the ankle joints at a constant 90° angle and thus essentially eliminated sway-related ankle joint proprioception. When eyes were closed and the platform rotated in exact proportion to body sway, vestibular cues became the most relevant sensory stimuli.

Before discussing the organization of postural responses in young children, we would like to summarize the results obtained in studies using the platform paradigm in adults. Nashner (1977), Nashner and Woollacott (1979), and Woollacott and Keshner (1984) report that platform movements cause body sway and activate a stereotypical sequential organization of muscle responses on the body surface opposite to the direction of the sway. Thus, for instance, for a backward translation of the platform causing forward sway, the stretched gastrocnemius muscle is activated at 90 to 100 ms, followed by hamstrings and trunk extensor muscles (see Figure 2). According to Nashner and McCollum (1985), this distal-to-proximal temporal organization is the most efficient for returning the body's center of mass to its original position. Other experiments investigating the importance of a variety of sensory inputs in the control of posture supported the hypothesis that proprioceptive information from the ankle level is primarily responsible for triggering these postural responses (Nashner, 1976).

Later research has expanded our understanding of the synergic organization of muscles contributing to posture control by exploring neck and trunk muscles' responses to platform perturbations. In addition to the responses radiating upward from the ankle joint, early (100 ms) responses occur in the neck muscles on the body surface opposite to that of the leg muscle activation (Woollacott & Keshner, 1984). The latencies of these upper body responses were unaffected by manipulating visual cues. However, when vestibular inputs were reduced (by rotating the platform around the ankle joint axis, which caused maximal ankle but minimal head movement), these neck muscle responses occurred significantly less often, leading to the conclusion that they may be activated via vestibular or neck proprioceptive inputs rather than ankle joint proprioceptors. However, the literature disagrees about the latency of vestibular postural responses. Interestingly, under these conditions the response pattern initiated in the lower leg musculature ascends beyond the upper leg and trunk to the neck muscles on the same side of the body, with increasing delays in onset latency (Woollacott & Keshner, 1984).

ANTERIOR SWAY – STANDING
adult

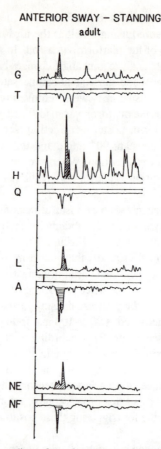

**Figure 2**  Surface EMG recordings of muscle responses of a standing adult to posterior platform translation causing forward sway (one trial). The two muscles recorded from each body segment are grouped together, with the flexor muscle inverted. The line indicates the onset of platform movement. Time marks are at 135-ms intervals.

When similar platform translations were given while adults were seated on a stool instead of standing, directionally appropriate responses were seen in the muscles of the trunk. Thus for translations causing forward sway, the trunk extensor muscles were activated, bringing the center of mass back to its original position. Neck muscles were also activated but in a variable manner. In the majority of cases, the neck extensor muscles were also activated at a slightly longer latency, consistent with the concept of a synergic response radiating upward from the base of support. However, occasionally neck flexors were also activated at early latencies, perhaps in response to vestibular or neck proprioceptive stimulation. In addition, the temporal organization of these responses showed a high variability between subjects, as opposed to the consistency seen in response to perturbations while standing (see Figure 3). This result may

ANTERIOR SWAY — SITTING

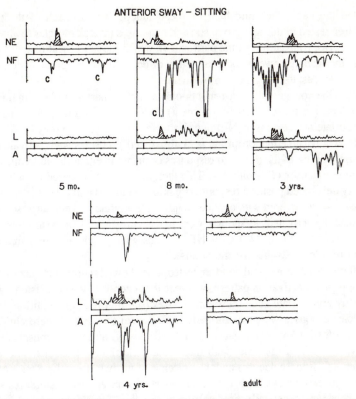

**Figure 3**   Surface EMG recordings of muscle responses of individuals in each age group to posterior platform translations while seated. Responses are represented as indicated in Figure 2.

be due to the easier balance requirements of the task (broader base of support and lower position of center of gravity).

The following section will describe postural responses of seated and standing children to movements of the support surface. Because children in the youngest age groups tested were often in transitional phases in learning to sit and stand independently, considerable intersubject variability existed. For this reason, their response patterns will be examined individually. We believe that this will elucidate the maturational trends in the development of the posture control system.

## POSTURAL RESPONSES IN CHILDREN

### Sitting

The youngest children we tested (4 to 5 months old) were unable to sit independently and therefore were tested in an infant seat. Though the seat supported the back, the child held the head independently. Each of the three children tested in this age group showed responses in neck muscles to anterior or posterior translations of the platform on which the infant seat rested. However, the responses were not consistently directionally appropriate in compensating for destabilizing head movement.

When the youngest child, a 4-month-old, was given posterior platform translations (causing forward head movement) under normal visual conditions, the appropriate neck extensor (NE) muscles were activated during only 60% of the trials, whereas the inappropriate neck flexor (NF) muscles were activated the remaining 40% of the time. No responses occurred in either the abdominal (A) or trunk extensor (TE) muscles. This lack of reaction appeared to indicate a poorly developed postural response organization in this child. However, when the eyes were covered with opaque goggles, NE muscles, to our surprise, were consistently activated. Responses were in the same latency range as those seen in the adults (117 ± 32 ms for NE muscles with no vision, compared to a mean of 136 ± 24 ms for the adults).

Of the two 5-month-old children tested, one showed repeated instances of an inappropriate activation pattern, whereas the second showed consistent directionally appropriate neck muscle responses (see Figure 3). In addition, trunk muscle responses were occasionally activated in the first of these children. For platform movements causing backward sway, abdominal muscles were activated 40% of the time, with mean latencies of 118 ± 26 ms. The wide variety of response patterns and the presence of many trials with no response in trunk muscles with eyes open do not support the concept that postural response synergies are genetically predetermined and thus functional independent of experience with stabilizing the center of mass. This initial inconsistency could indicate the presence of a trial-and-error learning period in the development of directionally specific postural responses in infants, during which the precise mapping of sensory inputs onto postural musculature takes place. The anatomical pathways may be genetically prewired but require experience to be activated. However, as mentioned earlier, in the 4-month-old consistent directionally appropriate neck muscle responses became apparent when vision was removed. Possibly the proprioceptive activation of postural responses becomes functional prior to that of the visual system but is dominated by visual inputs when they are available under normal visual conditions.

In contrast to the youngest age group of children tested while seated, the three children 8 to 14 months old who could sit independently showed clear directionally specific neck and trunk muscle responses characterized by low variability in onset latency (see Figure 3 and Table 1). This was also true for the group of 2- to 3-year-olds (Figure 3 and Table 1). As previously noted for adult responses, variability between subjects was observed in the pattern of temporal sequencing beginning from the base of support and moving upward. The temporal coupling of neck and trunk muscles thus does not seem to be

## Table 1

### Muscle Response Latencies for Platform Translations, Seated (in ms)

| | Neck Extensor | Trunk Extensor | Neck Flexor | Abdominal |
|---|---|---|---|---|
| Translations Causing Anterior Sway | | | | |
| 4–6 months | 141 ± 38 | NR | 209 ± 24 | 139 ± 49 |
| 8–14 months | 117 ± 38 | 109 ± 13 | NR | 117 ± 38 |
| 2–3 years | 132 $N$ = 1<br>NR = 1 | 115 ± 10 | NR | NR |
| Adults | 136 ± 24 | 130 ± 21 | 123 ± 25 | 144 ± 33 |
| Translations Causing Posterior Sway | | | | |
| 4–6 months | 123 ± 3 | NR | 122 ± 40 | 118 $N$ = 1 |
| 8–14 months | 123 ± 61 | NR | 158 ± 28 | 153 ± 26 |
| 2–3 years | 127 $N$ = 1 | NR | 137 ± 18 | 131 ± 5 |
| Adults | 117 ± 20 | 123 ± 13 | 121 ± 19 | 114 ± 25 |

*Note.* NR = no response; $N$ = number of subjects.

as critical to balance control while sitting, as is the temporal coupling of the leg and trunk muscles while standing.

As in the younger age group, postural responses were also activated by platform movements when the children's eyes were covered with opaque goggles. Figure 4 shows an example of responses of a 5-month-old and an 8-month-old to platform translations causing anterior sway with eyes covered. Note that in the example, the responses are even bigger than with eyes open (see Figure 3).

## Standing

The three children in the 8- to 14-month-old age group represented the full range of stages seen in learning to stand, from no experience in independent stance (8 months) through minimal experience (10 months), and finally to 1-1/2 months experience in stance and walking (14 months). As we saw in the children of the youngest age group tested while seated, these children showed an increase in response organization with age and experience standing. The 8-month-old (lightly supported at the waist by the mother as an aid in standing) showed *no* responses to platform movements causing anterior or posterior sway. Leg,

sitting − closed

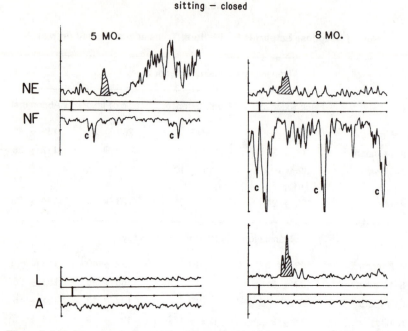

**Figure 4**  Muscle responses of seated 5- and 8-month-old children to posterior platform translations (anterior sway) with vision removed. Note that responses are still present. Time marks are
at 135-ms intervals.

trunk, and neck muscles were either tonically active or showed no response at
all. Thus, we observed lack of postural responses and lack of voluntary control
of leg muscles in stance. However, possibly in this younger child the support
given by the mother reduced the effect of the platform movement sufficiently
to prevent the stretch of the ankle musculature.

The 10-month-old showed appropriate responses in the gastrocnemius (G)
muscle during 40% of the platform movements causing anterior sway. They were
activated at very short, monosynaptic reflex latencies (53 ± 11 ms). Upper leg
muscles were activated in only one trial. Trunk and neck muscles were activated
in the majority of trials but were not consistently directionally appropriate. The
oldest child (the 14-month-old) showed directionally appropriate responses in
the leg muscles during all of the platform movements, at longer latencies consistent
with those seen in the adult. G latencies for anterior sway were 109 ± 24 ms;
tibialis anterior (TA) mean latencies for posterior sway were 161 ± 9 ms (see
Table 2). Neck and trunk responses, though often present, were not consistently
organized in the temporal sequence seen in the adult.

Thus, for the development of postural responses during standing (in this age
group) we see a clear increase in both the level of activation and the consistency

**Table 2**

**Muscle Response Latencies for Platform Translations, Standing (in ms)**

| | Translations Causing Anterior Sway | | | | | | | |
|---|---|---|---|---|---|---|---|---|
| | NF | NE | A | TE | Q | H | TA | G |
| 14 months | 30 ± 8 (n = 2) | 141 ± 15 | 96 n = 1 NR | 150 ± 32 | 96 n = 1 NR | a | 114 ± 45 | 109 ± 26 N = 1 |
| 2–3 years | 125 ± 21 (NR = 1S) | 150 ± 13 (NR = 2S) | 139 ± 46 (NR = 2S) | 173 ± 13 | 150 ± 52 | 160 ± 30 | 131 ± 24 (NR = 2S) | 109 ± 8 |
| 4–6 years | 122 ± 37 (NR = 1S) | 164 ± 19 (NR = 2S) | 125 ± 38 (NR = 2S) | 165 ± 20 (NR = 1S) | 181 ± 5 (NR = 4S) | 136 ± 26 (NR = 1S) | 168 ± 21 | 99 ± 5 (NR = 1S) |
| 7–10 years | 104 ± 16 | 153 ± 18 | 111 ± 16 | 161 ± 27 | 159 ± 24 | 137 ± 13 | 140 ± 30 | 96 ± 10 |
| Adults | 101 ± 5 | 131 ± 25 | 101 ± 13 | 131 ± 10 | 125 ± 20 | 120 ± 8 | 110 ± 7 | 91 ± 8 |

(Cont.)

**Table 2 (Cont.)**

Translations Causing Posterior Sway

| | NF | NE | A | TE | Q | H | TA | G |
|---|---|---|---|---|---|---|---|---|
| 14 months | 143 ± 53 | 45 n = 1<br>136 ± 36<br>(N = 2) | NR | 123 ± 10 | 164 ± 26 | [a] | 173 ± 18 | 107 (N = 1) |
| 2–3 years | 140 ± 7 | 116 ± 7 | 156 ± 16 | 94 ± 3 | 150 ± 16 | 196<br>(N = 1) | 102 ± 3 | 145 ± 26 |
| 4–6 years | 161 ± 35<br>(NR = 1S) | 131 ± 43 | 144 ± 33 | 165 ± 32 | 148 ± 29 | 141 ± 47 | 110 ± 10 | 111 ± 8 |
| 7–10 years | 155 ± 18 | 126 ± 12 | 153 ± 10 | 99 ± 10 | 146 ± 23 | 125 ± 40 | 100 2 19 | 140 ± 29 |
| Adults | 123 ± 34 | 102 ± 11 | 127 ± 9 | 149 ± 39 | 120 ± 17 | 99 ± 16 | 96 ± 17 | 148 ± 43 |

*Note.* NR = no response; S = subject; N = number of subjects; n = number of trials.
[a] Not recorded.

of organization of response patterns. This increase coincides with onset of voluntary use of the muscles in standing, with the youngest child showing no responses; the middle child showing proprioceptive monosynaptic reflexes; and the oldest child, with experience standing, showing consistently correct long latency responses in muscles of the leg, but less consistently organized responses in muscles of the trunk and neck (see Table 2).

The children in the 18-month- to 3-year-old age group showed clearly organized leg muscle responses to postural perturbations while standing. In previous studies (Forssberg & Nashner, 1982) and our first experiment (Shumway-Cook & Woollacott, 1985), children in this age group demonstrated the same distal-to-proximal muscle activation pattern as seen in adults. However, postural responses were consistently larger in amplitude and also longer in duration than those seen in the adult. The postural responses often overcompensated for platform induced sway and thus produced greater body oscillation than in the older children tested. In addition to the activation of the appropriate agonist muscles, which were effective in returning the center of gravity to its normal position, the children showed a large degree of activation of the antagonist leg muscles at a slightly longer latency. This reaction may be required to compensate for the large initial agonist muscle responses, or it may be due to a simple lack of refinement of the children's muscle response pattern.

One characteristic of postural muscle responses in adults is the propensity toward a relatively fixed amplitude ratio between muscles in a synergic grouping. Whereas amplitude of electromyograph responses can vary from trial to trial, the relationship between the amplitudes of distal and proximal leg muscles within a synergy remains relatively constant. The children in this group also demonstrated a low variability of muscle response amplitude ratios for the leg muscles, suggesting a tight coupling of proximal and distal leg muscle synergists (Shumway-Cook & Woollacott, 1985).

More recent studies (Woollacott et al., 1985) have analyzed the responses of children's trunk and neck muscles to platform movements. The development of the early secondary response synergy in the upper body musculature, which was described previously for adults, appears to occur later than the leg muscles response synergy. Thus the 2-1/2-year-old showed responses in the trunk musculature on only 20% of the trials. Early responses were apparent in neck flexor muscles during perturbations causing anterior sway but were never present in neck extensors in response to posterior sway. When we examined the number of trials in which neck flexor muscle responses were elicited in the 2- to 3-year-old age group in response to anterior sway, we found that they occurred 58% of the time, as opposed to occurring in 84% of the trials in the adult age group. When the neck flexor responses did appear, they occurred at approximately the same latency as in the adults (2- to 3-year-olds: 125 $\pm$ 21 ms; adults: 101 $\pm$ 5 ms) (see Table 2). However, trunk extensor and neck extensor muscles showed longer latencies in this age group than in the adults.

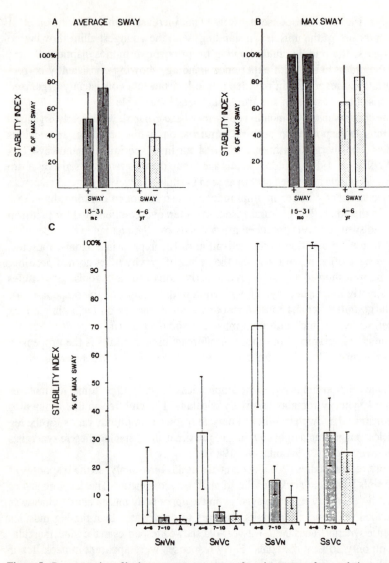

**Figure 5**   Representation of body sway as a percentage of maximum sway for translations causing anterior (+) and posterior (−) sway. A. 15 to 31 months; B. 4 to 6 years (from Shumway-Cook & Woollacott, 1985); C. Representation of body sway (as a percentage of maximum sway) under four sensory conditions, during 5 s of stance. SnVn: normal ankle joint somatosensory and normal visual inputs; SnVc: normal ankle joint somatosensory inputs with eyes closed; SsVn: ankle joint somatosensory inputs minimized, vision normal; SsVc: ankle joint somatosensory inputs minimized with eyes closed. Three age groups compared: 4 to 6 years, 7 to 10 years, and adults (from Shumway-Cook & Woollacott, 1985).

The amplitude of body sway during platform perturbations is a critical indicator of stability. Figures 5a and b graphically indicate the extent of body sway seen during postural perturbations in a group of 18- to 31-month-olds and 4- to 6-year-olds (Shumway-Cook & Woollacott, 1985). The stability index represents the amount of body sway in response to platform motion (a belt at the hips was connected to a potentiometer via a rod); a score of 100 indicates loss of balance. As can be seen in the figure, in response to platform translations children aged 18 to 31 months swayed on average close to their limits of stability (Figure 5a). In addition, they often reached their limit of stability (lost balance) during a trial (Figure 5b). This observation is consistent with the developmental literature indicating that stability is poor in young children. Though onset latencies were similar to those of adults for leg muscle responses, young children showed an increased rate of sway (Forssberg & Nashner, 1982). This faster rate of sway would result in the young child more often reaching the maximum point of stability prior to recovery resulting from the onset of muscle responses.

Initial experiments analyzing the onset latency and variability of the leg muscle responses of 4- to 6-year-olds (Shumway-Cook & Woollacott, 1985) revealed a startling finding. The 4- to 6-year-olds appeared to regress in their postural response organization, in that leg postural response synergies were more variable as compared to the 15- to 31-month-olds, 7- to 10-year-olds, or adults. In this age group, postural synergies were less consistent regarding both onset latencies and timing relationships between distal and proximal leg muscle synergists than in any other age groups. Whereas 15- to 31-month-old children exhibited onset latencies comparable to 7- to 10-year-olds and adults, latencies in the 4- to 6-year-old children were both significantly *slower* and more *variable* ($p < .01$). In addition, the 4- to 6-year-olds showed a significant delay in the activation of proximal leg muscle synergists. This diminished temporal coupling between leg muscles resulted biomechanically in a buckling of the knee joint during compensatory body sway. This phenomenon was not observed in the adult group, where compensation for platform-induced sway occurred primarily at the ankle with minimal angular displacement of hip and knee. The activation of the proximal leg muscles of the 4- to 6-year-olds was apparently not rapid enough to minimize the inertial lag associated with the mass of the thigh and trunk (Shumway-Cook & Woollacott, 1985).

The 4- to 6-year-old group also showed a significantly greater variability of the ratio of amplitudes of responses of the distal and proximal leg muscles than seen in the other age groups tested ($p < .05$), suggesting that proximal and distal leg synergists were less tightly coupled.

Our recent studies (Woollacott et al., 1985) analyzing the responses of trunk and neck muscles in these children support the earlier indication of high variability in response patterns. Under normal visual conditions for anterior sway perturbations, neck flexor muscle responses occurred less often in the 4- to 6-year-olds (22% of the trials) than in the 2- to 3-year-olds (54% of the trials) or the adults (84% of the trials). When present they were more variable (122 $\pm$ 37 ms) than the other age groups tested (2- to 3-year-olds: 125 $\pm$ 21 ms; adults: 101 $\pm$ 5 ms) (see Table 2). Trunk extensor muscle responses were also significantly longer in latency when compared to the adults ($p < .05$). However, despite this variability the 4- to 6-year-olds swayed less during platform movements than the younger age group (see Figures 5a and b).

The 7- to 10-year-old age group analyzed in our first study exhibited postural responses that were essentially like those seen in the adult age group in that no significant differences were seen in onset latency, variability, temporal coordination, or amplitude ratios between muscles within the leg synergy. However, in our second study measuring upper body muscle responses, the 7- to 10-year-olds showed longer onset latencies in neck and trunk extensor muscles when compared to the adult group. For trunk muscles, these differences were significant ($p < .025$), whereas for neck muscles differences fell just short of significance ($p < .057$). Thus we can conclude that leg muscle responses are essentially mature in this age group, whereas upper body responses do not completely mature until at least 10 years of age (see Table 2).

## Postural Responses With Eyes Closed

Removal of visual inputs (with opaque goggles) during horizontal platform movements had differing effects in the various age groups tested. In all age groups (including the youngest, which were tested in an infant seat), postural responses remained when visual cues were absent. In fact, in the youngest child tested (4 months), consistent, directionally appropriate neck muscle responses were present only when vision was removed. This observation suggests that removal of vision heightened the sensitivity of the system to proprioceptive and/or vestibular cues.

Figure 6 shows the differences in latency between eyes open/closed conditions for NF and G muscles for the 2- to 3-year-olds, 4- to 6-year-olds and adults for platform movements causing anterior sway. As mentioned previously, adults showed no significant differences in latency of these responses for the two conditions (Woollacott & Keshner, 1984). However, the 2- to 3-year-olds showed a reduction in the latency of neck muscle responses from 125 $\pm$ 21 ms to 98 $\pm$ 17 ms with an additional increase in the frequency of neck muscle monosynaptic reflexes. No changes were observed in the frequency of longer latency responses in the neck muscles (54% of the trials both with eyes open and closed). G response latencies were unchanged (open: 109 $\pm$ 8 ms; closed:

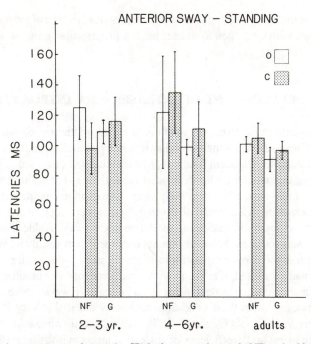

**Figure 6** Average response latency ($\pm$ *SD*) in the appropriate neck (NF) and ankle (G) muscle in response to translations causing anterior sway. Responses are shown for conditions with vision present (O) and absent (C) for three age groups: 2 to 3 years, 4 to 6 years, and adults.

116 $\pm$ 16 ms) in this same group of 2- to 3-year-olds; however, an increase in monosynaptic reflex occurrence did take place (open: 19%; closed: 30% of trials).

The 4- to 6-year-olds exhibited greater variability in neck and leg muscle latencies. With vision removed they showed an increase in the frequency of postural responses in neck muscles from activation in 22% of the trials to activation in 58% of the trials.

What is the significance of either a reduction in response latency or an increase in the frequency of occurrence of monosynaptic and longer latency responses when vision is removed? Either effect implies that visual cues are not required to activate postural responses in any of the age groups tested and, moreover, that removal of these cues actually increases the sensitivity of the system to the remaining proprioceptive and vestibular cues. The slight reduction in latency of neck muscle responses and increased number of monosynaptic reflexes in the 2- to 3-year-olds with vision removed could imply that vision is normally dominant in this age group, and that a shift occurs from the use of longer latency visual inputs with eyes open to shorter latency proprioceptive inputs with eyes closed.

## THE DEVELOPMENT OF INTERSENSORY INTEGRATION

The use of platform rotations instead of horizontal translations to perturb balance offers a unique way of testing the ability to adapt postural responses to changing task conditions. Platform rotations, like translations, cause ankle rotations and concomitant stretch to the ankle joint musculature, but without a shift in the center of mass and significant body sway. Thus, ankle joint proprioceptive inputs associated with *horizontal* platform movements are congruent with visual and vestibular inputs in indicating moderate body sway. Ankle joint inputs associated with rotations, however, are not congruent with visual and vestibular inputs because the former inputs indicate strong sway, whereas the latter are only minimally activated, if at all. In adults, platform rotations produce postural responses in the stretched ankle muscles on initial trials. However, these responses are *destabilizing* under these conditions and are attenuated to very low levels within three to five trials (Nashner, 1976). Thus, dorsiflexing ankle rotations can be used to test (a) the efficiency of ankle joint inputs in isolation in producing postural responses and (b) the ability to attenuate postural responses, when needed due to changing task conditions.

Three children between 15- and 31-months-old were tested with dorsiflexing rotational platform perturbations. Though monosynaptic reflexes were occasionally observed under these conditions, none of the subjects showed consistent longer latency postural responses in gastrocnemius (G) and hamstrings (H).

By 3 years of age the children exhibited normal, longer latency response synergies in leg muscles to platform rotations. The 4- to 6-year-olds also exhibited these responses. In addition, two thirds of the 4- to 6-year-old children tested showed attenuation of inappropriate responses, but not within the three to five trials seen in the adults. They required, instead, the exposure to 10 to 15 trials before response attenuation occurred. The 7- to 10-year-olds showed adult-like adaptation.

A second approach was also used to test children's ability to adapt to altered sensory conditions and to determine the way in which changes in sensory inputs affect postural muscle responses. Children were asked to stand quietly for 5 s under four different sensory conditions that progressively decreased sensory inputs relevant for balance control, until only vestibular inputs remained: (a) somatosensory ankle joint and visual inputs normal (SnVn); (b) somatosensory ankle joint inputs normal and eyes closed (SnVc); (c) ankle joint inputs minimized by rotating the platform in direct relationship to body sway but vision normal

(SsVn); and (d) ankle joint inputs minimized with eyes closed (SsVc). Performance was measured by determining body sway as a percent of theoretical maximum sway for each child, with 100% indicating loss of balance. The mean performance level for each of the conditions is indicated in Figure 5c for the 4- to 6-year-olds, 7- to 10-year-olds, and adults (the youngest children would not tolerate the altered conditions without crying). Even under normal stance conditions (SnVn) the 4- to 6-year-olds swayed significantly more than the older children or adults. With eyes closed (SnVc) their stability decreased further, but they retained balance. However, when the support surface was rotated with body sway, thus keeping the ankle joint at approximately 90° (SsVn), the 4- to 6-year-olds were greatly destabilized, and one lost balance. In the final condition in which ankle joint inputs were minimized and eyes were closed, leaving only vestibular cues to aid in balance (SsVs), four of the five children in this age group lost balance, whereas none of the older children or adults needed assistance to maintain their stability (Shumway-Cook & Woollacott, 1985).

Thus, we conclude that children under 7 years of age are unable to balance efficiently when both somatosensory and visual cues are removed and only vestibular cues remain to control stability. The 4- to 6-year-olds showed progressively decreasing stability as they lost redundant sensory inputs for postural control. They also appeared to have difficulty in shifting from the use of ankle joint somatosensory cues to visual cues when ankle joint inputs were made incongruent with body sway (by rotating the platform with body sway). This may also indicate the 4- to 6-year-olds' inability to resolve intersensory conflict during postural control.

## POSTURAL AND VOLUNTARY RESPONSE INTEGRATION

In preliminary experiments designed to determine the relationship between postural and voluntary muscle responses in children, standing children were asked to push or pull on a handle in response to the illumination of a set of brightly colored lights (Shumway-Cook, 1983). Muscle responses were recorded from the biceps (B) and triceps (T) of the upper arm, as well as the gastrocnemius (G) and tibialis anterior (TA) muscles of the leg. Experiments on four normal adults with this apparatus confirmed previous findings (Cordo & Nashner, 1982), showing preparatory postural activity in the G muscle prior to the B muscle for all pull trials and in TA prior to T for all push trials (see Figure 7). Four of the five children in the 4- to 6-year-old group showed postural preparatory activity in all trials, whereas the last child showed preparatory activity in 80% of the trials. This suggests that by 4 to 6 years of age, integration of the voluntary and postural systems is essentially mature and character-

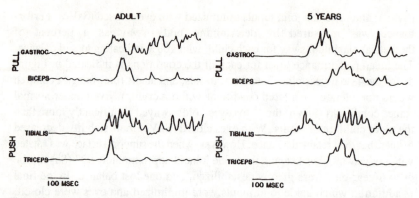

**Figure 7**   Responses of leg and arm muscles during reaction time arm movements (push or pull) while standing. Note that postural activity in the leg precedes prime mover activity in the arm, indicating feed-forward postural control in both the 5-year-old and adult.

ized by a feed-forward control process that anticipates instability associated with voluntary movement and minimizes it by the mean of preparatory postural responses.

Future experiments will test postural-voluntary response integration abilities in younger children, in order to determine if the integration of responses in the two systems is present as soon as postural synergies are initially stabilized at the age of 2 to 3 years.

## APPLICATIONS TO TEACHING MOTOR SKILLS

One of the clear principles emerging from balance control studies is the existence of at least three phases in the development of postural control. In children first learning to stand, there is a dominance of visual cues in triggering postural responses, and these responses tend to be short in latency and relatively stereotyped. The age of 4 to 6 years marks a clear transitional phase, with responses becoming longer in latency and increasingly variable. By the third phase (7 to 10 years), the leg responses have attained adult-like characteristics, though upper body responses continue to evolve during this period.

During the period of time when children acquire and refine basic locomotor skills (18 months to 3 years), they seem to rely primarily on visual information. The apparent regression in the postural organization that occurs between 4 and 6 years of age may be associated with a time period during which the child learns to integrate visual, proprioceptive, and vestibular cues in the maintenance of balance. We hypothesize that children progressively expand their reliance on sensory information to systems other than the visual system. The fine tuning of the regulation of stance and posture resulting from this calibration of the three systems appears to be a mandatory stage in learning, and it leads to adult-like postural control in which responses are both short in latency and adaptive to changing task conditions.

The age range of 4 to 6 years appears to be a time of sensory exploration for the child, in which information from all sensory modalities is used in order to practice flexible alterations between different modalities. Motor skill training at this age level should stress playfulness and exposure to a wide range of conditions. Educators should let the child explore and discover a variety of solutions to the task that must be mastered. If children are put under great pressure to perform to a criterion, they could revert to more primitive but more accurate visually guided behaviors, if these behaviors are relevant to the given situation. On the other hand, they might simply become discouraged and give up. In either case, they would never progress beyond a rigid stereotyped pattern of movement or widen their range of motor skills. This lack of flexibility could also occur in situations in which children are restricted to practicing one form of closed skill activity. Such a condition would possibly restrict the chances to encounter sufficiently varied situations to accommodate optimally to changing conditions and to develop diversified abilities.

Our knowledge that children rely predominantly on visual information for balance control at early ages, together with the awareness that they are unable to shift successfully to the use of other modalities when visual inputs are erroneous, should guide our expectations of children's motor performance under the age of 4 to 6 years. The constraint of visual guidance certainly limits motor learning capabilities. The educator should keep this in mind and focus on situations aimed to help the child master the treatment of visual information and the basic skills. These observations and suggestions are consistent with those presented by Bressan and Woollacott (1982) in reformulating Jewett's model for a prescriptive paradigm for sequencing instruction in physical education. In this formulation, the first construction subphase in motor skill acquisition consists initially of a playful level of learning where the performer attempts to sort out the kinds of sensory information gathered from the visual, vestibular, and somatosensory systems that pertain to the skill or task to be learned.

We hope that the physical educator continues to emphasize this early subphase of skill acquisition in the child's early years of development (possibly through age 7), rather than stress the skill subphase of stabilization. This approach would ensure that children have adequate practice in a wide range of sensory circumstances to gain the appropriate integrational and strategic ability to move on to the final learning subphase of differentiation where they learn to vary, improvise, and even compose new subroutines for action.

## Acknowledgments

This research was supported by grants from the Medical Research Foundation of Oregon and NIH (#R23-A605317-01) to M. Woollacott, The Medical Research

Foundation of Paris to B. Debû, and NIH Training Grant 1-T32-MH17148-01
to A. Shumway-Cook.

## REFERENCES

Belenkii, V.E., Gurfinkel, V.S., & Paltsev, R.I. (1967). On the elements of
voluntary movement control. *Biofizika,* **12**, 135–141.

Bower, T.G.R. (1972). Object perception in infants. *Perception,* **1**, 15–30.

Bower, T.G.R. (1974). *Development in infancy.* San Francisco: W.H. Freeman.

Bower, T.G.R., Broughton, J.M., & Moore, M.K. (1970). The coordination
of visual and tactual input in infants. *Perception and Psychophysics,* **8**, 51–53.

Bressan, E., & Woollacott, M. (1982). A prescriptive paradigm for sequencing
instruction in physical education. *Human Movement Science,* **1**, 155–175.

Butterworth, G. (1982). The origins of auditory-visual perception and visual
proprioception in human development. In R. Walk & H. Pick (Eds.), *Intersensory perception and sensory integration* (pp. 37–70). New York: Plenum
Press.

Butterworth, G., & Hicks, L. (1977). Visual proprioception and postural stability
in infancy: A developmental study. *Perception,* **6**, 255–262.

Cordo, P.J., & Nashner, L.M. (1982). Properties of postural adjustments
associated with rapid arm movements. *Journal of Neurophysiology,* **47**, 287–
302.

Forssberg, H., & Nashner, L. (1982). Ontogenetic development of posture
control in man: Adaptation to altered support and visual conditions during
stance. *Journal of Neuroscience,* **2**, 545–552.

Gahery, Y., & Massion, J. (1981). Coordination between posture and movement. *Trends in Neuroscience,* **4**, 199–202.

Horak, F.B., Esselman, P., Anderson, M.E., & Lynch, M.K. (1984). The
effects of movement velocity, mass displaced and task certainty on associated
postural adjustments made by normal and hemiplegic individuals. *Journal
of Neurology, Neurosurgery, and Psychiatry,* **47**, 1020–1028.

Lee, D.N., & Aronson, E. (1974). Visual proprioceptive control of standing in
human infants. *Perception and Psychophysics,* **15**, 529–532.

Lee, W.A. (1980). Anticipatory control of postural and task muscles during
rapid arm flexion. *Journal of Motor Behavior,* **12**, 185–196.

Legallet, E., & Gahery, Y. (1980). Influence of a diagonal postural pattern
on parameters of movement and associated postural adjustment in the cat.
*Experimental Brain Research,* **40**, 35–44.

Massion, J., & Gahery, Y. (1979). Diagonal stance in quadrupeds: A postural support for movement. In R. Granit & O. Pompeiano (Eds.), *Progress in brain research: Reflex control of posture and movement* (Vol. 50, pp. 219–226). Amsterdam: Elsevier.

Nashner, L.M. (1976). Adapting reflexes controlling human posture. *Experimental Brain Research, 26,* 59–72.

Nashner, L.M. (1977). Fixed patterns of rapid postural responses among leg muscles during stance. *Experimental Brain Research, 30,* 13–24.

Nashner, L.M., & McCollum, G. (1985). The organization of human postural movements: A formal basis and experimental synthesis. *Behavior Brain Science, 8,* 135–172.

Nashner, L.M., & Woollacott, M. (1979). The organization of rapid postural adjustments of standing humans: An experimental-conceptual model. In R.E. Talbot & D.R. Humphrey (Eds.), *Posture and movement* (pp. 243–257). New York: Raven Press.

Shumway-Cook, A. (1983). *Developmental aspects of postural control in normal and Down's syndrome children.* Unpublished doctoral dissertation, University of Oregon, Eugene.

Shumway-Cook, A., & Woollacott, M.H. (1985). The growth of stability: Postural control from a developmental perspective. *Journal of Motor Behavior, 17,* 131–197.

Traub, M.M., Rothwell, J.C., & Marsden, C.D. (1980). Anticipatory postural reflexes in Parkinson's disease and other akinetic-rigid syndromes and in cerebellar ataxia. *Brain, 103,* 393–412.

Woollacott, M., Debû, B., & Mowatt, M. (1985, April). *The development of balance control in children: Sensorimotor integration.* Paper presented at the annual meeting of the North American Society for the Psychology of Sport and Physical Activity, New Orleans.

Woollacott, M., & Keshner, E. (1984). Upper body responses to postural perturbations in man. *Neuroscience Abstracts, 10,* 635.

Yonas, A. (1981). Infants' responses to optical information for collision. In R. Aslin, J. Alberts, & M. Petersen (Eds.), *Development of perception: Vol. 2. The visual system* (pp. 313–334). New York: Academic Press.

# 11

# Motor Behavior and Psychosocial Correlates in Young Handicapped Performers

**Greg Reid**

The present chapter differs from others in this volume in that the principal focus is on a variety of theoretical issues as they pertain to subject populations rather than the usual analysis of a specific theoretical or empirical domain. As such, a range of motor behavior and psychosocial theories will be discussed, albeit rather briefly, because the emphasis is on individual differences and how these theories pertain to the motor performance of young handicapped individuals. These individuals are children who have difficulty participating in the culturally normative physical activities and sport typical of their age because of learning problems (mental retardation, learning disabilities, physical awkwardness, and autism).

In the last 20 years, the number of disabled youngsters participating in a variety of physical activities has increased dramatically. This point alone should encourage researchers to seek a better understanding of the role of physical activity and competition in the growth and development of disabled persons. Many disabled individuals, however, perform rather poorly compared with nondisabled peers. A single or obvious reason rarely exists for this discrepancy, but some of the most important factors will be advanced, primarily the motor learning correlates of handicapped performers and the motivational posture exhibited by some of them.

## A NOTE ON TERMINOLOGY

The word *handicapped* will be used synonymously with *disability* and *impairment*. However, the American Alliance for Health, Physical Education, and Recreation (AAHPER) (1971) and the World Health Organization (1980) have suggested a differentiation of these terms. *Impairment*, it is argued, should be restricted to denote a loss or abnormality in psychological, physiological, or anatomical structure or function. For example, an amputation is an impairment. A disability is any restriction in performing activities typical for an individual of a given age in his or her culture. A lower limb amputation is thus a disability for walking but not for typing. Finally, a handicap is viewed as a disadvantage for an individual resulting from an impairment or disability that prevents involvement within the person's capabilities. Handicaps may be internally imposed (e.g., "I am blind therefore I will not try to swim because it is impossible") or societally imposed (e.g., occupational restrictions despite competence) (McCarthy, 1984). For example, Buell (1982) has argued that blindness is a nuisance but should not be a handicap. In this sense, a handicap represents prejudice against the individual on the basis of imagined difficulties with an activity. Indeed, educators (Martin, 1974), psychologists (Asch, 1984), and movement specialists (Reid, 1979; Wade, Hoover, & Newell, 1983) have noted that a handicap, as an attitudinal prejudice imposed by an unknowing society, may be the most significant hurdle a person with an impairment must overcome.

The distinctions among impairment, disability, and handicap are not maintained for the present chapter because they have not been widely adopted in academic circles or by government agencies. However, the implications are much more important than a quibble of semantics. In fact, researchers should increase their productivity in this area where they have heretofore been silent and thereby help to reduce the stigma of special populations. Psychologists have not been as active with disabled persons as they might (Kahn, 1984). The following section will outline how current investigators of developmental physical activity might expand their research interests and contribute to our knowledge of young impaired performers.

## SPECIAL POPULATIONS: THEORY AND RESEARCH

Special populations have been used in research for three possible reasons: (a) to determine program effectiveness; (b) to generalize theory; and (c) to construct theory.

Researching program effectiveness refers to those investigations in which improving the lot of the subjects, rather than advancing theory per se, is the zeitgeist. Such studies *do* have a theoretical foundation, but the resulting data are limited to interpreting the effectiveness of an intervention rather than promoting a theoretical position.

As investigators develop a specific theory, they must assess the boundaries of generalization (Snow, 1979). Although this notion of generalizability is not new, the use of special populations to extend the boundaries of a theory is not commonplace. Asch (1984) has argued that "we need to know whether existing psychological theories and research methods can account for the experience of disabled people" (p. 533). Asch was concerned primarily with the psychological domain, but her statement should be considered more broadly. In other words, including disabled subjects in research designs will not only provide important extensions or limits to the theory itself but will also increase our understanding of the disability. Examples of theory generalization in the motor domain with special populations include work on Fitts' Law (e.g., Newell, Wade, & Kelly, 1979) and a developmental sequence of overarm throwing (Roberton & DiRocco, 1981).

Special populations may be fundamental to the very heart of research, theory construction. Vygotsky (1978) recognized this point in the 1920s. Of course, some theoretical stances have been designed to explain handicapped conditions (e.g., Fisher & Zeaman, 1973) without particular reference to nonhandicapped persons. However, what is the role of special populations for broader construction of theory? Roy (1978) and Kelso and Tuller (1981) invoked different theoretical explanations for apraxia but argued that the study of this movement disorder should aid our understanding of the intact motor system. Also, Bower (1981) has reviewed the special populations literature to argue that some infant behaviors seem maturationally determined rather than functions of experience. He points out that congenitally deaf youngsters will show the first phase of babbling, and congenitally blind children will "observe" and track their own hands moving to and fro. Finally, Campione and Brown (1978) have concluded from their work with the mentally retarded that the "hallmark of intelligence is the ability to generalize information from one situation to another and that this ability in turn depends upon effective 'executive control'" (p. 279).

The point has been made that special populations should be included in a wider range of experimental paradigms to increase the generality of established theory and to help build emerging theory. A caveat should be introduced, however. Consider the common procedure of blindfolding subjects to gain important information of the kinesthetic and proprioceptive systems. Arguably, these systems' function and contribution to motor control without vision may be different from their involvement when vision is available. This is a specific example of the general notion that what people "do" in normal circumstances differs from what they "can do" in abnormal circumstances (Newell & Barclay, 1982). Thus special populations may be important contributors to theory construction, but they should not be considered substitutes for established means.

## GUIDING THEORETICAL PERSPECTIVES

Newell (1985b) and Hoover and Wade (1985) have outlined the influences of three theoretical postures of psychology that have guided most of the motor skill acquisition research of the mentally retarded: (a) behavioral psychology, (b) information processing, and (c) ecological psychology. Their discussions, however, are germane to other special populations and are therefore being adapted in the present generic chapter.

### Behavioral Psychology

Behavioral or stimulus-response psychology was the major force in psychology during the first half of the 20th century and maintains its impact in special populations research today (Hoover & Wade, 1985). Motor skill acquisition was viewed as a chaining of discrete responses. Furthermore, the learner was considered to be rather passive, not strategically involved in the learning process. The independent variables chosen by the researchers were external to the subject. For example, motor skill acquisition by special populations was characterized by topics such as the influence of reinforcement, praise, or incentives (e.g., Auxter, 1969; Ellis & Distenfano, 1959) or mass versus distributed practice (e.g., Drowatzky, 1970).

Behavioral psychology was the birthplace of operant conditioning and behavior modification. Reinforcement, ignoring, punishment, and other behavior modification techniques remain influential in modern physical activity research with special populations. Particularly with lower functioning, multihandicapped individuals, these techniques are the prime means to promote exercise (e.g., Caouette & Reid, 1985; Stainbeck, Stainbeck, Wehman, & Spangler, 1983; Tomporowski & Ellis, 1984) and to acquire movement and leisure skills (e.g., Collier & Reid, in press). Although such studies reveal little about how learning occurs, behavioral principles will remain in vogue within the program effectiveness research scheme previously discussed.

### Information Processing

Information-processing psychology began to influence experimental psychology after World War II but had little impact upon skill acquisition in special populations until the late 1960s. This approach attempts to chronicle the various stages of information transmission between a stimulus input and a response outcome. Atkinson and Shiffrin (1968) outlined an information-processing model of human memory that became influential in special populations research. They proposed that memory could be distinguished by structures (short-term sensory store, short- and long-term store) that were permanent, unchanging components and by control processes (e.g., rehearsal) that were optional and selected at the individual's will. The control processes actively interacted with stimuli to ensure passage throughout the structural features. This model intrigued many researchers in mental retardation because the concept of structure, if specified, would relate to intelligence (Fisher & Zeaman, 1973) and thus be important in defining mental retardation. The structural versus process control distinction remains a popular heuristic although determining what is structure and what is process is sometimes difficult, and developmentalists now acknowledge that both structure and process will change, the former possibly less slowly than the latter (Butterfield, 1981; Campione & Brown, 1978; Newell, 1984).

## Ecological Psychology

The third and most recent theoretical influence of movement skills in special populations is that of ecological psychology. The ecological perspective is rooted in Gibson's (1979) direct perception theory. Gibson and his followers argue that environmental information that specifies use or affordance to the person is directly available in the optic array (to use visual perception as an example), and we need not invoke interpretations, evaluations, and other indirect processes that intervene between stimuli and the perceived. Such indirect processes characterize information processing. Furthermore, perception depends on the organism's needs and capabilities, and therefore it must be viewed as a function of both the perceiver and the environment.

Ecological psychology also addresses the degrees-of-freedom problem articulated by Bernstein (1967). He viewed coordination as the mastery of redundant degrees of freedom. Although overly simplistic, the joints of the body may be considered degrees of freedom potentially free to vary. Reducing their movement where appropriate in skill acquisition reduces the degrees of freedom.

The ecological approach to action unites and extends the notions of Gibson and Bernstein and argues that motor development can best be understood as a naturally developing system. It attempts to minimize the influence of cognition, which is so overriding in information processing. Theorists who have extended Gibson's and Bernstein's formulations distinguish between coordination, control, and skill (Kugler, Kelso, & Turvey, 1982). Newell's (1985a) use of the terms is likely to influence research with special populations. He asserts that coordination may be viewed as a set of relative motions, whereas control is defined by the scaling of the given relative motions. In this light, some descriptive data of special populations now exist (e.g., Beuter, 1984).

# MOTOR SKILL PERFORMANCE

The physical skills of the handicapped usually have been assessed by motor ability batteries that often combine performance and fitness items. This section will view the descriptive motor skill data with each disability group before discussing common themes and concerns.

## Mental Retardation

More motor performance data pertain to the mentally retarded than to any other special population. Also, major descriptive reviews have existed for a number of years (e.g., Bruininks, 1974; Rarick, 1973). Much of this work was influenced by the research of Rarick and colleagues who have shown that the factor structure of mildly retarded youngsters is similar to that of nonhandicapped groups (Dobbins & Rarick, 1975). Cross-sectional studies show that the change in performance with age is also similar to that of the nonhandicapped (Francis & Rarick, 1959; Rarick, Dobbins, & Broadhead, 1976). However, clear evidence from this work demonstrates that the retarded perform less well and with greater within- and between-subject variability than their more intellectually capable counterparts on measures of strength, power, throwing, balance, flexibility, jumping, and fine motor control. The retarded also are low in maximum oxygen uptake (Coleman, Ayoub, & Friedrich, 1976; Maksud & Hamilton, 1974), and they are burdened with excess body fat.

Although less work has been done with more severely retarded individuals, a relationship seems apparent between intellect and motor performance; moderately retarded groups usually score lower than mildly retarded groups (Londeree & Johnson, 1974). Yet, as one descends the intellectual ladder, assessment on standardized tests for comparative research becomes problematic because of accompanying sensory, behavioral, and orthopedic difficulties.

Individuals with Down's syndrome compose the largest clinical subcategory in mental retardation, and like other retarded persons they are less physically skilled than the nonhandicapped. The more interesting question is whether or not this group is different from subjects of equal mental age. The data are somewhat cloudy, and solid and consistent evidence that they are significantly unlike other retarded persons has not yet emerged (see reviews by Anwar, 1981; Henderson, 1985; Reid, 1985).

## Learning Disabilities and Physical Awkwardness

When they were initially identified as a group requiring special education intervention, children with learning disabilities were described as evidencing motor performance difficulties (e.g., Kephart, 1960). Bruininks and Bruininks (1977) systematically compared learning disabled and nondisabled youngsters on the

Bruininks-Osteretsky Test of Motor Proficiency. With the exception of their results on a response-speed subtest, the learning disabled group was inferior and more variable.

Children with learning disabilities are usually defined operationally for research by low and variable academic scores, particularly in reading. Some of these youngsters do not have a learning disability in the reading sense but are physically clumsy. Recently, therefore, physical educators have begun to recognize the clumsy child (e.g., Arnheim & Sinclair, 1980; Reid, 1982) as one who requires special attention regardless of any accompanying learning disability. In fact, future research should separate these two groups to determine their unique developmental patterns and physical activity needs. When physically awkward–learning disabled children are removed from the learning disabled group, what are the performance profiles of this latter group? Similarly, what are the meaningful differences between those physically awkward children who have a concomitant learning disability and those that do not? Also, distinguishable subgroups do appear within the clumsy child population (Dare & Gordon, 1970; Henderson & Hall, 1982). Much of the present research has confounded these conditions. Logically, movement specialists should begin with children with movement problems and look for subdivisions within that group, rather than start the same process with learning-disabled children and look for clumsy children.

A physically awkward child is defined as one who is unable to adequately perform culturally normative movements expected of his or her age but who is at least intellectually average and neurologically intact (Gubbay, 1975; Wall, 1982). Approximately 5 or 6% of the school-aged population may be clumsy (Keogh, Sugden, Reynard, & Calkins, 1979; Wall, 1982). These youngsters are identified by teachers and parents due to their ineptitude in motor performance; therefore, it is not surprising that a standardized test including measures of balance, ball skills, and manual dexterity differentiates clumsy from nonclumsy children (Henderson & Hall, 1982).

Most descriptions of physically awkward children have been clinical in nature. Their early motor development of sitting alone and walking may be delayed (Gordon & McKinlay, 1980). As they mature, they may have difficulties tying shoelaces, dressing, and writing. Furthermore, they usually dread physical education classes. Among the qualitative descriptors of these children are inconsistency, perseveration, mirroring, asymmetry, falling after performance, extraneous movements, excessive energy expenditure, inability to control force, and arrhythmical and inappropriate motor planning (Keogh et al., 1979; Haubenstricker, 1982; Henderson & Hall, 1982; Walton, Ellis, & Court, 1962). Although this profile paints a rather global motor deficit picture, detailed and comprehensive observation has suggested that these youngsters may adequately perform tasks that minimize body equilibrium adjustments, such as swimming or horseback riding (Gordon & McKinlay, 1980).

## Autism

Motor development in autistic children was considered normal in early reports (e.g., Kanner, 1943), but more recent evidence suggests otherwise. Ornitz, Guthrie, and Farley (1977) used a parent questionnaire report and concluded that autistic youngsters are slower than nonhandicapped infants in attaining the developmental milestones of the first year of life such as lifting the head, sitting, crawling, and walking. Furthermore, the differences appear to grow in the second 6 months of life.

Because the majority of autistic persons are also mentally retarded, comparisons between these groups on motor skill have been inevitable. DeMyer (1976) concluded from a study of perceptual and motor performances that autistic and mentally retarded children are similar on most motor items with the exception of ball skills, in which the autistic youngsters are particularly deficient. Reid, Collier, and Morin (1983) compared autistic children (mean age 10.2 years) and adolescents (mean age 16.6 years) on a wide range of anthropometric, motor performance, and fitness items. In general, the two groups of autistic subjects differed little with the exception of height and weight; they were inferior when compared to previously established norms of mentally retarded and nonhandicapped groups.

Poor motor performance associated with autism was corroborated by Morin and Reid (1985). However, in this study, relatively high-functioning autistic adolescents were chosen ($n = 8$, mean IQ $= 66$), and they were compared to age and IQ-matched peers. This was deemed necessary to ferret out the relative contribution of mental retardation to motor performance in autism. Although the numbers were low, the two groups were generally quite similar. Researchers tentatively concluded that the poor motor skills shown by autistic learners may be largely a function of mental retardation rather than autism per se.

## THE NEED FOR MORE DESCRIPTIVE DATA

Despite seemingly abundant data describing the motor performance of special populations, particularly the mentally retarded, much needed research is still essentially descriptive in nature. First, some special population groups have only recently come to the attention of movement specialists. These include the autistic, the severely mentally retarded, and paradoxically, the physically awkward. A paucity of movement-related information exists about these conditions and their subgroups. Do the physically awkward really perform at par when body equilibrium adjustments are minimized? If the study of Morin and Reid (1985) was replicated with more subjects, would the poor performance of autistic individuals be primarily a function of retardation?

Second, almost all of the descriptive data available is quantitative in nature (how fast, how close). Certainly from a practitioner's point of view, qualitative knowledge about the placement of feet in an overarm throw or the use of arms in a long jump is more valuable teaching information because many types of movement can produce the same score (DiRocco & Roberton, 1981). Some qualitative descriptions of special populations have been published (e.g., Morin & Reid, 1985; Ulrich, 1983), and with the development of valid and reliable qualitative tests (e.g., Mosher & Schutz, 1983; Ulrich, 1985) this practice should become more commonplace. Detailed descriptions must consider the person-environment synergy from the ecological perspective (Davis, 1984). Also, assessing the relative motions of the disabled as suggested by ecological advocates (Newell, 1985b), although initially descriptive, is linked to a theoretical account of coordination (Kugler, Kelso, & Turvey, 1982). It will also be informative to determine the relationship between quantitative and qualitative measures. Some special populations are possibly characterized by greater quantitative than qualitative deficits (Roberton & DiRocco, 1981).

A third need is increased longitudinal research with special populations. Virtually all data, even in the comparatively rich area of retardation, is cross-sectional in nature. Both Reid et al. (1983) with autistic children and Roberton and DiRocco (1981) with retarded subjects noted a period of apparent arrested motor development. Henderson (1985) has suggested that Down's syndrome youngsters may demonstrate periods of rapid progress and at other times no apparent development. These observations can only be clarified and understood by longitudinal analyses.

## EXPLAINING INDIVIDUAL DIFFERENCES

The reasons for handicapped-nonhandicapped differences in motor behavior usually remain unanswered by descriptive research. The following factors may contribute to such wide individual differences: (a) characteristics of the condition, (b) anthropometric constraints, (c) opportunities and practice, (d) information processing, and (e) motivational attitude.

### Characteristics of the Condition

The condition itself can influence motor performance sometimes rather directly and at other times indirectly. With deaf children, vestibular deficits appear to be a relatively direct factor in explaining balance problems, whereas language deprivation may be an indirect influence (Wiegersma & Velde, 1983). Furthermore, if testing occurs in a novel environment, autistic subjects, who are characterized as being resistant to change, may not perform optimally. Finally, if a mentally retarded subject does not understand test protocol, his or her results may indicate intellectual rather than motor retardation.

## Anthropometric Constraints

Anthropometric constraints may also contribute to motor performance. In some groups of special populations, for example, people with Down's syndrome, the individuals are distinct in stature. Down's syndrome children are not only shorter than age expectations, but their limbs are disproportionately short (Thelander & Pryor, 1966). Indeed, mentally retarded persons tend to be shorter and weigh less than chronological-aged peers (Bailit & Whelan, 1967; Rundle & Sylvester, 1973). When adjustments for body size are made, some performance deficits are eliminated (Dobbins, Garron, & Rarick, 1981). The contribution of anthropometric status to performance is a vastly underresearched area and may prove to be powerful in explaining developmental differences (see Newell, 1984 for a more complete discussion of this issue).

## Opportunity and Practice

Although current estimates are not available, in the 1960s special populations such as the mentally retarded were believed to have less opportunity to engage in physical activity. Institutions clearly may restrict the movement opportunities of the incarcerated (Henderson, 1985). Not surprisingly, therefore, their performance on motor tasks suffers when compared to noninstitutionalized peers. If any group of children is overprotected because of their handicap, their performance will likely be below what might be expected. Thus the initial performance level demonstrated by handicapped youth is not likely to be an accurate predictor of learning potential.

## Information Processing

The information-processing perspective was attractive to special education researchers because many viewed it as a vehicle to determine specific deficits. They assumed that once the area of processing difficulty was determined, remedial procedures could be implemented. To highlight the area of deficiency, comparative research was necessary. In the area of mental retardation investigators recognized that simply demonstrating retarded-nonhandicapped differences on a single task, even one designed to access a particular process, would do little more than redefine mental retardation (Baumeister, 1967). Such data would be fundamentally correlational with nothing inherent to suggest a causal relationship between mental retardation and specific cognitive deficits because nonspecific factors such as motivation, incentive, and attentiveness could be equally plausible explanations (Stanovich, 1978). The tact adopted was a search for interactions (Baumeister, 1967; Detterman, 1979; Stanovich, 1978).

   An interaction was necessary before a specific deficit could be inferred (Stanovich, 1978). If the subject groups (e.g., retarded-nonhandicapped) were similar at one level of the independent variable, the nonspecific factors such as attention could be ruled out as potential explanations of the differences found. The difference, or deficit, could then be argued to be indigenous to the subject group.

The search for specific information-processing deficits by mentally retarded subjects on motor tasks has implicated the following difficulties: attentiveness (Kirby, Nettelbeck, & Thomas, 1979); perceptual processing in time to acquire information (Nettelbeck & Lally, 1979); decision processing such as linking a stimulus with the appropriate response (Brewer, 1978; Brewer & Nettelbeck, 1979); response capacity and organization (Sugden & Gray, 1981); coincident timing (Wade, Newell, & Hoover, 1982); and short-term memory (Reid, 1980b). All stages of processing movement-related information have seemed problematic for retarded subjects. These findings lead Newell (1985b) to conclude that information processing has been just another description of mentally retarded persons' motor performance. That the mentally subnormal might be rather globally defective in terms of cognitive processing has been echoed by others (Henderson, 1985; Nettelbeck & Brewer, 1981; O'Connor & Hermelin, 1981).

As investigators have tried to identify specific structural deficits, they have also employed a training study approach that is guided more toward identifying control processes that might be responsible for slow-learning children's depressed performance. Most of this research has occurred outside the motor domain and is admirably reflected in a number of review papers (Belmont & Butterfield, 1977; Brown, Bransford, Ferrara, & Campione, 1983; Borkowski & Cavanaugh, 1979; Campione, Brown, & Ferrara, 1982). In essence, retarded youngsters were regarded as rather passive learners who seldom interacted intentionally to remember or learn material. Similar conclusions have been reached in the learning disability literature (Hagen, Barclay, & Schwethelm, 1982). In the area of memory, researchers began to teach children a number of strategic techniques such as rehearsal, organizational modifications, and elaboration. Dramatic improvements often occurred. The retarded seemed able to become strategic learners. In the motor skills domain, both Reid (1980a) and Horgan (1983) have shown that encouraging retarded subjects to employ memory techniques improved their recall on simple tasks.

When investigators attempted to demonstrate the generality of the newly learned strategic techniques on novel tasks, their findings were generally disappointing (Brown et al., 1983; but see Borkowski & Cavanaugh, 1979 for an alternative interpretation). They viewed transfer as a major stumbling block and dependent on some "executive control" that functioned to select, monitor, and check strategic control. Executive control is essentially metacognition (Flavell & Wellman, 1977), and the training of these skills is attracting considerable investigation (Brown et al., 1983; Campione et al., 1982). Motor development theorists have not fully treated metacognition, although strategies and executive control with special populations should see considerable work in the future.

Some have interpreted the success of the strategic intervention schemes to prove that no structural limit exists for the mentally retarded. However, Campione et al. (1982) have countered that a specific structural deficit has simply not yet been found. Also, despite the improvements via strategic instruction shown by the mentally retarded, they do not consistently perform at nonhandicapped levels. Indeed, not to accept some notion of structural limitations in retarded individuals is to assume training will eliminate retardation, which "begs the question: Why are retarded persons retarded?" (Ellis, Deacon, & Woolridge, 1985, p. 401).

Finally, Newell's (1985b) implication that researchers should abandon the information-processing perspective for retarded citizens might be premature. The emerging knowledge base (Chi, 1978; Wall, McClements, Bouffard, Findlay, & Taylor, 1985) and strategic intervention outgrowths of information processing (e.g., Reid, in press) may provide considerable explanatory power in determining the difficulties experienced by retarded persons with physical skills. Also, the search for specific processing deficits may prove more successful for other disability groups such as the physically awkward.

## Motivational Attitude

The importance of motivation in an achievement context has attracted considerable attention from developmental (Dweck & Elliot, 1983) and special population (Ruble & Boggiano, 1980) perspectives. The learned helplessness construct has been commonly invoked to explain the amotivational attitude with which many disabled individuals approach achievement situations. When an individual does not perceive a relationship between his or her responses and subsequent reinforcement, a state of helplessness appears to emerge. The individual who feels that nothing he or she does is adequate will eventually stop trying and will drop out in a voluntary physical activity context.

The conceptualization of learned helplessness has been advanced by Weiner's (1974) model of attribution (see also Horn, 1987). He argues that people explain success or failure on the basis of unstable/stable factors and internal/external factors. Ability and task difficulty are relatively stable factors, whereas effort and luck are unstable factors that may vary from trial to trial, task to task. Effort and ability are internal factors, whereas luck and task difficulty are external factors. Under normal circumstances, success is probably attributed to internal factors of ability and effort, and failure is explained by external reasons. Repeated failure, however, is attributed to stable factors (Dweck, 1980). Helplessness attributed to internal-stable factors (e.g., ability) has a more debilitating effect than that caused by internal-unstable factors (e.g., effort) (Canino, 1981).

Most children in special education have a long history of failure. Mildly retarded youngsters are not usually identified until they have difficulties in school. Learning-disabled children are defined in many school districts as scoring 1 year or more below expectations on achievement tests. Failure is almost a prerequisite to remediation. In a physical activity setting in which failure is open for all to observe, particularly pronounced and early attributions to lack of ability may occur. MacMillan and Keogh (1971) highlighted the possibility that special populations may attribute failure to internal factors. When the experimenter manipulated whether or not children completed a task, nonretarded children used excuses that blamed others, whereas retarded children consistently blamed themselves.

Although some literature supports the notion that internal attributions for failure are common in special populations, some also illustrates that individuals with learning or emotional problems possess an external orientation (Dudley-Marling, Snider, & Tarver, 1982; Lawrence & Winchell, 1975). The externality is a result rather than cause of long-term failure (Dudley-Marling et al., 1982). An external orientation refers to a loss of control over one's destiny and is conceptually related to outer-directedness (Balla & Zigler, 1979). Such individuals feel they don't control their performance and show minimal independence in learning, always being reliant upon others for orientation. Furthermore, according to the cognitive evaluation theory of intrinsic motivation (Deci & Ryan, 1980), an external locus of causality will reduce one's intrinsic motivation toward an activity, a major goal in promoting physical recreation for handicapped children (Lewko, 1978).

Griffin and Keogh (1982) have developed a model of movement confidence that views confidence as an individual's feeling of adequacy in a movement context. Movement confidence is viewed as both a consequence and mediator in movement. Confidence as a mediator affects three aspects of participation: choice, performance, and persistence. Consistent with the aforementioned explanations of intrinsic motivation, attribution and learned helplessness, the consistently failing performer may choose not to participate. If participation occurs, the lack of movement confidence will likely reduce information-processing effectiveness and will be characterized by a lack of persistent effort. Movement confidence is also viewed as a consequence of a personal evaluation in relation to the demands of a movement situation. The Griffin and Keogh model may prove to be an effective vehicle to view the psychosocial theories mentioned in this section within a physical activity milieu because it revolves primarily around movement, not academic achievement. Despite the amotivational nature of special populations suggested earlier in this section, experience indicates that many people with handicaps are highly motivated performers and may be more successful in movement than in other achievement contexts. An individual approach is obviously implied.

Evidence shows that children with learning problems are likely to score lower on tests purporting to measure self-concept and peer status (Balla & Zigler, 1979; Bruininks, 1978) and that physical prowess is positively related to aspects of social development (Smoll, 1974). Furthermore, physically awkward children admit that their friends make fun of them, they are not well liked, and they are often sad (Cratty, Ikeda, Martin, Jennett, & Morris, 1970). Recent research by Shaw, Levine, and Belfer (1982) linked clumsiness and academic learning problems. They showed that children who were physically awkward and academically behind expectations despite average IQ had significantly lower self-esteem than children who were "simply" having academic difficulties. Thus, ineptitude in movement itself can be a problem to the emotional status of a child and an additional burden when in concert with learning problems. Self-esteem is a multifaceted concept, and changes in movement proficiency should not be seen as a panacea. However, skilled movement may be an important variable in minimizing the debilitating influence of academic learning problems (see also the chapter by Weiss in this volume).

Vallerand and Reid (1985) have attempted to highlight remedial implications for the failure-prone performer from the models presented in this section. The first and most obvious way to enhance the perception of competence is to provide the performer with success experiences. The task-analysis approach evident in contemporary curriculum models for special populations is an example. Second, positive verbal feedback on performance should enhance intrinsic motivation through enhanced perceived competence (Vallerand & Reid, 1984) if the feedback is linked to competence. Third, physical activity specialists should consider attributional retraining (e.g., Dweck, 1975) as part of the intervention plan to break the learned helpless, internal (lack of ability) cycle. Learners must be helped to realistically sense when lack of success is due to task difficulty and effort rather than ability. For example, with retarded subjects, Hoffman and Weiner (1978) showed that only success experiences followed by attributions to ability enhanced future performance. Thus, learners must begin to take credit for success. Finally, success experiences should be linked with stress-coping strategies. If a student encounters a situation that is unlike the rather isolated and comforting clinic environment, he or she must learn to use available resources to deal with the stress rather than assume a helplessness/low self-esteem attitude (Stevens & Pihl, 1982). This should increase the transfer from a clinical setting and may heighten self-concept (Stevens & Pihl, 1982). Of course this latter recommendation dovetails nicely with the strategy-metacognition training elucidated under information processing.

## SUMMARY AND CONCLUSIONS

Generally, from a motor performance perspective the handicapped differ undeniably from the nonhandicapped. Yet longitudinal analyses of motor skill development and qualitative observational and kinematic measures are neglected research strategies. In other words, the emergence of this motor performance deficit has not been adequately detailed. Such data would have obvious practical import as well as theoretical significance. As noted earlier, the use of handicapped subjects, particularly the physically awkward, in research designs is essential to theoretical development.

How can the often poor motor performance of special populations be explained? Possible reasons adumbrated here include characteristics of the condition itself, anthropometric constraints, opportunities and practice, information processing, and lack of motivation. What is not clear from the literature are the limits of these restrictions. To what extent can information processing or motivational difficulties be ameliorated? And how will such a development influence performance? Again, determining the trainability of these limitations will have practical and theoretical significance.

Information processing, as noted, has been a popular approach to movement research. What has been learned, however, has been at the expense of knowledge about learning because information processing is primarily performance oriented. *How* do handicapped persons acquire a motor skill? Do they follow the same principles as the nonhandicapped? Dunn (1983) has stated, "Handicapped students learn in accordance with the same learning principles as normal students, only usually slower" (p. 64), whereas Sherrill (1983) has argued, "It is naive to say that severely handicapped children develop fitness and learn motor skills in the same way as do the mildly and moderately impaired" (p. 74). These statements may not be as polemic as they appear, for each author may have implicit assumptions about what is learning the same or differently. Investigators should explicitly articulate these assumptions in future research. Presumably, demonstrations of aptitude by teaching interactions (Snow, 1979) are required to support notions that handicapped children learn differently. Although handicapped and nonhandicapped performers differ in some obvious ways, the explanations and limits to these differences should continue to be explored.

## REFERENCES

American Alliance for Health, Physical Education, and Recreation. (1971, September). A clarification of terms. *Journal of Health, Physical Education, and Recreation*, pp. 63–68.

Anwar, F. (1981). Motor function in Down's Syndrome. In N.R. Ellis (Ed.), *International review of research in mental retardation* (Vol. 10, pp. 107–138). New York: Academic Press.

Arnheim, D., & Sinclair, W. (1980). *The clumsy child* (2nd ed.). St. Louis, MO: Mosby.

Asch, A. (1984). The experience of disability: A challenge for psychology. *American Psychologist, 39*, 529–536.

Atkinson, R.E., & Shiffrin, R.M. (1968). Human memory: A proposed system and its control process. In K.W. Spence & J.T. Spence (Eds.), *The psychology of learning and motivation* (Vol. 2, pp. 189–195). New York: Academic Press.

Auxter, D. (1969). Effects of reinforcement on motor learning and retention by the mentally retarded. *Perceptual and Motor Skills, 29*, 99–104.

Bailit, H.L., & Whelan, M.A. (1967). Some factors related to size and intelligence in the institutionalized mentally retarded population. *Journal of Pediatrics, 71*, 897–909.

Balla, D., & Zigler, E. (1979). Personality development in retarded persons. In N.R. Ellis (Ed.), *Handbook of mental deficiency* (2nd ed., pp. 143–168). Hillsdale, NJ: Lawrence Erlbaum.

Baumeister, A.A. (1967). Problems in comparative studies of mental retardation and normals. *American Journal of Mental Deficiency, 71*, 869–875.

Belmont, J.M., & Butterfield, G.C. (1977). The instructional approach to developmental cognitive research. In R.V. Kail, Jr., & J.W. Hagen (Eds.), *Perspectives on the development of memory and cognition* (pp. 437–481). Hillsdale, NJ: Lawrence Erlbaum.

Bernstein, N. (1967). *The coordination and regulation of movements*. New York: Pergamon Press.

Beuter, A. (1984). Describing multijoint coordination: Preliminary investigation with nonhandicapped, cerebral palsied, and elderly individuals. *Adapted Physical Activity Quarterly, 1*, 105–111.

Borkowski, J.G., & Cavanaugh, J.C. (1979). Maintenance and generalization of skills and strategies by the retarded. In N.R. Ellis (Ed.), *Handbook of mental deficiency* (2nd ed., pp. 569–617). Hillsdale, NJ: Lawrence Erlbaum.

Bower, T.G.R. (1981). *Development in infancy* (2nd ed.). San Francisco: W.H. Freeman.

Brewer, N. (1978). Motor components in the choice reaction time of mildly retarded adults. *American Journal of Mental Deficiency, 82*, 565–572.

Brewer, N., & Nettelbeck, T. (1979). Speed and accuracy in the choice reaction time of mildly retarded adults. *American Journal of Mental Deficiency, 84*, 55–61.

Brown, A.L., Bransford, J.D., Ferrara, R.A., & Campione, J.C. (1983). Learning, remembering and understanding. In P.H. Mussen (Ed.), *Handbook of child psychology* (4th ed., Vol. 4, pp. 77–166). New York: Wiley & Sons.

Bruininks, R.H. (1974). Physical and motor development of retarded persons. In N.R. Ellis (Ed.), *International review of research in mental retardation* (Vol. 7, pp. 209–261). New York: Academic Press.

Bruininks, V.L. (1978). Peer status and personality characteristics of learning disabled and nondisabled students. *Journal of Learning Disabilities, 11*, 29–34.

Bruininks, V.L., & Bruininks, R.H. (1977). Motor proficiency of learning disabled and nondisabled students. *Perceptual and Motor Skills, 44*, 1131–1137.

Buell, C.E. (1982). *Physical education and recreation for the visually handicapped*. Washington, DC: AAHPERD.

Butterfield, E.C. (1981). Testing process theories of intelligence. In M.P. Friedman, J.P. Das, & N. O'Connor (Eds.), *Intelligence and learning* (pp. 277–296). New York: Plenum Press.

Campione, J.C., & Brown, A.L. (1978). Toward a theory of intelligence: Contributions from research with retarded children. *Intelligence, 2*, 279–304.

Campione, J.C., Brown, A.L., & Ferrara, R.A (1982). Mental retardation and intelligence. In R.J. Sternberg (Ed.), *Handbook of human intelligence* (pp. 392–490). New York: Cambridge University Press.

Canino, F.J. (1981). Learned-helplessness theory: Implications for research in learning disabilities. *Journal of Special Education, 15*, 471–484.

Caouette, M., & Reid, G. (1985). Increasing the work output of severely retarded adults on a bicycle ergometer. *Education and Training of the Mentally Retarded, 20*, 296–304.

Chi, M.T.H. (1978). Knowledge structures and memory development. In R. Siegler (Ed.), *Children's thinking: What develops?* (pp. 73–96). Hillsdale, NJ: Lawrence Erlbaum.

Coleman, A.E., Ayoub, M.M., & Friedrich, D.W. (1976). Assessment of the physical work capacity of institutionalized mentally retarded males. *American Journal of Mental Deficiency, 80*, 692–695.

Collier, D., & Reid, G. (in press). *A comparison of two models designed to teach autistic children a motor task*. Manuscript submitted for publication.

Cratty, B.J., Ikeda, N., Martin, M.M., Jennett, C., & Morris, M. (1970). *Movement activities, motor ability and the education of children*. Springfield, IL: C.C. Thomas.

Dare, M.T., & Gordon, N. (1970). Clumsy children: A disorder of perception and motor organization. *Developmental Medicine and Child Neurology, 12*, 178–185.

Davis, W.E. (1984). Motor ability assessment of populations with handicapping conditions: Challenging basic assumptions. *Adapted Physical Activity Quarterly, 1*, 125–140.

Deci, E.L., & Ryan, R.M. (1980). The empirical exploration of intrinsic motivational processes. In L. Berkowitz (Ed.), *Advances in social psychology* (Vol. 13, pp. 39–80). New York: Academic Press.

DeMyer, M.K. (1976). Motor, perceptual-motor, and intellectual disabilities of autistic children. In L. Wing (Ed.), *Early childhood autism* (pp. 169–193). Oxford, England: Pergamon Press.

Detterman, D.K. (1979). Memory in the mentally retarded. In N.R. Ellis (Ed.), *Handbook of mental deficiency* (2nd ed., pp. 727–760). Hillsdale, NJ: Lawrence Erlbaum.

DiRocco, R., & Roberton, M.A. (1981, March). Implications of motor development research: The overarm throw in the mentally retarded. *The Physical Educator*, pp. 27–31.

Dobbins, D.A., Garron, R., & Rarick, G.L. (1981). The motor performance of educable mentally retarded and intellectually normal boys after covariate control for differences in body size. *Research Quarterly for Exercise and Sport, 52*, 1–8.

Dobbins, D.A., & Rarick, G.L. (1975). Structural similarity of the motor domain of normal and educable retarded boys. *Research Quarterly, 46*, 447–456.

Drowatzky, J.N. (1970). Effects of mass and distributed practice schedules upon the acquisition of pursuit rotor tracking by normal and mentally retarded subjects. *Research Quarterly, 41*, 342–348.

Dudley-Marling, C.C., Snider, V., & Tarver, S.G. (1982). Locus of control and learning disabilities: A review and discussion. *Perceptual and Motor Skills, 54*, 503–514.

Dunn, J.M. (1983). Physical activity for the severely handicapped: Theoretical and practical considerations. In R.L. Eason, T.L. Smith, & F. Caron (Eds.), *Adapted physical activity* (pp. 63–73). Champaign, IL: Human Kinetics.

Dweck, C.S. (1975). The role of expectations and attributions in the alleviation of learned helplessness. *Journal of Personality and Social Psychology, 31*, 674–685.

Dweck, C.S. (1980). Learned helplessness in sport. In C.H. Nadeau, W.R. Halliwell, K.M. Newell, & G.C. Roberts (Eds.), *Psychology of motor behavior and sport—1979* (pp. 1–11). Champaign, IL: Human Kinetics.

Dweck, C.S., & Elliot, E.S. (1983). Achievement motivation. In P.H. Mussen (Ed.), *Handbook of child psychology* (Vol. 4, pp. 643–691). New York: Wiley & Sons.

Ellis, N.R., Deacon, J.R., & Woolridge, P.W. (1985). Structural memory deficits of mentally retarded persons. *American Journal of Mental Deficiency, 89*, 393–402.

Ellis, N.R., & Distenfano, M.K. (1959). Effects of verbal urging and praise upon rotary pursuit performance in mental defectives. *American Journal of Mental Deficiency, 64*, 486–490.

Fisher, M.A., & Zeaman, D. (1973). An attention-retention theory of retardates discrimination learning. In N.R. Ellis (Ed.), *International review of research in mental retardation* (Vol. 6, pp. 169–256). London: Academic Press.

Flavell, J.H., & Wellman, H.M. (1977). Metamemory. In R.V. Kail, Jr. & J.W. Hagen (Eds.), *Perspectives on the development of memory and cognition* (pp. 3–33). Hillsdale, NJ: Lawrence Erlbaum.

Francis, R.J., & Rarick, G.L. (1959). Motor characteristics of the mentally retarded. *American Journal of Mental Deficiency,* **63**, 292–311.

Gibson, J.J. (1979). *The ecological approach to visual perception*. Boston: Houghton Mifflin.

Gordon, N., & McKinlay, I. (Eds.). (1980). *Helping clumsy children*. Edinburgh: Churchill Livingstone.

Griffin, N.S., & Keogh, J.F. (1982). A model for movement confidence. In J.A.S. Kelso & J.E. Clark (Eds.), *The development of movement control and coordination* (pp. 213–236). New York: Wiley & Sons.

Gubbay, S. (1975). Clumsy children in normal schools. *The Medical Journal of Australia,* **1**, 233–236.

Hagen, J.W., Barclay, C.R., & Schwethelm, B. (1982). Cognitive development of the learning-disabled child. In N.R. Ellis (Ed.), *International review of research in mental retardation* (Vol. 11, pp. 1–41). New York: Academic Press.

Haubenstricker, J.L. (1982, May). Motor development in children with learning disabilities. *Journal of Physical Education, Recreation and Dance,* pp. 41–43.

Henderson, S. (1985). Motor skill development. In D. Lane & B. Stratford (Eds.), *Current approaches to Down's syndrome*.(pp. 187–218). London: Holt, Rinehart & Winston.

Henderson, S., & Hall, D. (1982). Concomitants of clumsiness in young school children. *Developmental Medicine and Child Neurology,* **24**, 448–460.

Hoffman, J., & Weiner, B. (1978). Effects of attributions for success and failure on the performance of retarded adults. *American Journal of Mental Deficiency,* **82**, 449–452.

Hoover, J.H., & Wade, M.G. (1985). Motor learning theory and mentally retarded individuals: A historical review. *Adapted Physical Activity Quarterly,* **2**, 228–252.

Horgan, J.S. (1983). Mnemonic strategy instruction in coding, processing and recall of movement-related cues by mentally retarded children. *Perceptual and Motor Skills,* **57**, 547–557.

Horn, T.S. (1987). The influence of teacher-coach behavior on the psychological development of children. In D. Gould & M.R. Weiss (Eds.), *Advances in pediatric sport sciences: Vol. 2. Behavioral issues* (pp. 121–142). Champaign, IL: Human Kinetics.

Kahn, A.S. (1984). Perspectives on persons with disabilities. *American Psychologist, 39,* 516–517.

Kanner, L. (1943). Autistic disturbances of affective contact. *The Nervous Child, 2,* 217–250.

Kelso, J.A.S., & Tuller, B. (1981). Toward a theory of apraxtic syndromes. *Brain and Language, 12,* 224–245.

Keogh, J.F., Sugden, D.A., Reynard, C.L., & Calkins, J.A. (1979). Identification of clumsy children: Comparisons and comments. *Journal of Human Movement Studies, 5,* 32–41.

Kephart, N.C. (1960). *The slow learner in the classroom.* Columbus, OH: C.E. Merrill.

Kirby, N.H., Nettelbeck, T., & Thomas, P. (1979). Vigilance performance of mildly mentally retarded children. *American Journal of Mental Deficiency, 84,* 184–187.

Kugler, P.N., Kelso, J.A.S., & Turvey, M.T. (1982). On the control and coordination of naturally developing systems. In J.A.S. Kelso & J.E. Clark (Eds.), *The development of movement control and coordination* (pp. 5–78). New York: Wiley & Sons.

Lawrence, E., & Winchell, J.E. (1975). Loss of control: Implication for special education. *Exceptional Children, 42,* 483–490.

Lewko, J.H. (1978). Significant others and sport socialization of the handicapped child. In F.L. Smoll & R.E. Smith (Eds.), *Psychological perspectives in youth sports* (pp. 249–277). Washington, DC: Hemisphere.

Londeree, B., & Johnson, L. (1974). Motor fitness of TMR vs EMR and normal children. *Medicine and Science in Sport, 6,* 247–252.

MacMillan, D.L., & Keogh, B.K. (1971). Normal and retarded children expectancy for failure. *Developmental Psychology, 4,* 343–348.

Maksud, M.G., & Hamilton, L.H. (1974). Physiologic response of EMR children to strenuous exercise. *American Journal of Mental Deficiency, 79,* 32–38.

Martin, E.W. (1974). Some thoughts on mainstreaming. *Exceptional Children, 41,* 150–153.

McCarthy, E.A. (1984). Is handicap external to the person and therefore "man made"? *British Journal of Mental Subnormality, 30,* 3–7.

Morin, D., & Reid, G. (1985). A quantitative and qualitative assessment of autistic individuals on selected motor tasks. *Adapted Physical Activity Quarterly, 2,* 43–55.

Mosher, R., & Schutz, R. (1983). The development of a test of overarm throwing: An application of generalizability theory. *Canadian Journal of Applied Sport Sciences,* **8**, 1–8.

Nettelbeck, T., & Brewer, N. (1981). Studies of mild mental retardation and timed performance. In N.R. Ellis (Ed.), *International review of research in mental retardation* (Vol. 10, pp. 61–106). New York: Academic Press.

Nettelbeck, T., & Lally, M. (1979). Age, intelligence and inspection time. *American Journal of Mental Deficiency,* **83**, 398–401.

Newell, K.M. (1984). Physical constraints to development of motor skills. In J.E. Thomas (Ed.), *Motor development during childhood and adolescence* (pp. 105–120). Minneapolis, MN: Burgess.

Newell, K.M. (1985a). Coordination, control and skill. In D. Goodman, I. Franks, & R. Wilberg (Eds.), *Differing perspectives in motor control.* Amsterdam: North Holland.

Newell, K.M. (1985b). Motor skill acquisition and mental retardation: Preview of traditional and current orientations. In J.E. Clark & J.H. Humphrey (Eds.), *Current selected research in motor development* (pp. 183–192). Princeton, NJ: Princeton Book Company.

Newell, K.M., & Barclay, C.R. (1982). Developing knowledge about action. In J.A.S. Kelso & J.E. Clark (Eds.), *The development of movement control and co-ordination* (pp. 175–212). New York: Wiley & Sons.

Newell, K.M., Wade, M.G., & Kelly, T.M. (1979). Temporal anticipation of response initiation in retarded persons. *American Journal of Mental Deficiency,* **84**, 289–296.

O'Connor, N., & Hermelin, B. (1981). Intelligence and learning: Specific and general handicap. In M.P. Friedman, J.P. Das, & N. O'Connor (Eds.), *Intelligence and learning* (pp. 51–65). New York: Plenum Press.

Ornitz, E.M., Guthrie, D., & Farley, A.J. (1977). The early development of autistic children. *Journal of Autism and Childhood Schizophrenia,* **7**, 208–229.

Rarick, G.L. (1973). Motor performance of mentally retarded children. In G.L. Rarick (Ed.), *Physical activity: Human growth and development* (pp. 227–256). New York: Academic Press.

Rarick, G.L., Dobbins, D.A., & Broadhead, G.D. (1976). *The motor domain and its correlates in educationally handicapped children.* Englewood Cliffs, NJ: Prentice-Hall.

Reid, G. (1979). Mainstreaming in physical education: The concept and its implications. *McGill Journal of Education,* **14**, 367–377.

Reid, G. (1980a). The effects of memory strategy instruction in the short term motor memory of the mentally retarded. *Journal of Motor Behavior*, **12**, 221–227.

Reid, G. (1980b). Overt and covert rehearsal in short-term memory of mentally retarded and nonretarded persons. *American Journal of Mental Deficiency*, **85**, 69–77.

Reid, G. (1982). Physical education for the learning disabled student: An update. *Learning Disabilities Quarterly*, **5**, 190–193.

Reid, G. (1985). Physical activity programming. In D. Lane & B. Stratford (Eds.), *Current approaches to Down's syndrome* (pp. 219–241). London: Holt, Rinehart & Winston.

Reid, G. (in press). The trainability of motor processing strategies with developmentally delayed performers. In M. Wade & H.T.A. Whiting (Eds.), *Themes in motor development*. Amsterdam: North Holland.

Reid, G., Collier, D., & Morin, B. (1983). Motor performance of autistic individuals. In R.L. Eason, T.L. Smith, & F. Caron (Eds.), *Adapted physical activity* (pp. 201–218). Champaign, IL: Human Kinetics.

Roberton, M.A., & DiRocco, P. (1981). Validating a motor skill sequence for mentally retarded children. *American Journal of Corrective Therapist*, **35**, 148–154.

Roy, E.A. (1978). Apraxia: A new look at an old syndrome. *Journal of Human Movement Studies*, **4**, 191–210.

Ruble, N.N., & Boggiano, A.K. (1980). Optimizing motivation in an achievement context. In B.K. Keogh (Ed.), *Advances in special education* (Vol. 1, pp. 183–238). Greenwich, CT: JAI Press.

Rundle, A.T., & Sylvester, P.E. (1973). Evaluation of physical maturity in adolescent mentally retarded boys. *Journal of Mental Deficiency Research*, **17**, 89–96.

Shaw, L., Levine, M.D., & Belfer, M. (1982). Developmental double jeopardy: A study of clumsiness and self-esteem in children with learning problems. *Developmental and Behavioral Pediatrics*, **3**, 191–196.

Sherrill, C. (1983). Pedagogy in the psychomotor domain for the severely handicapped. In R.L. Eason, T.L. Smith, & F. Caron (Eds.), *Adapted physical activity* (pp. 74–88). Champaign, IL: Human Kinetics.

Smoll, F.L. (1974). Motor impairment and social development. *American Corrective Therapy Journal*, **28**, 4–6.

Snow, R.G. (1979). Theory and method for research on aptitude processes. In R.J. Sternberg & D.K. Detterman (Eds.), *Human intelligence* (pp. 105–137). Norwood, NJ: Ablex.

Stainback, S., Stainback, N., Wehman, P., & Spangler, L. (1983). Acquisition and generalization of physical fitness exercise in three profoundly retarded adults. *The Journal of The Association for the Severely Handicapped*, **8**, 47–55.

Stanovich, K.E. (1978). Information processing in mentally retarded individuals. In N.R. Ellis (Ed.), *International review of research in mental retardation* (Vol. 9, pp. 29–60). New York: Academic Press.

Stevens, R., & Pihl, R.O. (1982). The remediation of the student at risk for failure. *Journal of Clinical Psychology*, **38**, 298–301.

Sugden, D.A., & Gray, S.M. (1981). Capacity and strategies of educationally subnormal boys on serial and discrete tasks involving movement speed. *British Journal of Educational Psychology*, **51**, 77–82.

Thelander, H.E., & Pryor, H.B. (1966). Abnormal patterns of growth and development in mongolism. *Clinical Pediatrics*, **5**, 493–501.

Tomporowski, P.D., & Ellis, N.R. (1984). Preparing severely and profoundly mentally retarded adults for tests of motor fitness. *Adapted Physical Activity Quarterly*, **1**, 158–163.

Ulrich, D.A. (1983). A comparison of the qualitative motor performance of normal, educable, and trainable mentally retarded. In R.L. Eason, T.L. Smith, & F. Caron (Eds.), *Adapted physical activity* (pp. 219–225). Champaign, IL: Human Kinetics.

Ulrich, D.A. (1985). *Test of gross motor development*. Austin, TX: Pro-Ed.

Vallerand, R.J., & Reid, G. (1984). On the causal effects of perceived competence on intrinsic motivation: A test of cognitive evaluation theory. *Journal of Sport Psychology*, **6**, 94–102.

Vallerand, R.J., & Reid, G. (1985). Intrinsic motivation: Implications for teaching the failure-prone performer. Unpublished manuscript.

Vygotsky, L.S. (1978). *Mind in society*. Cambridge, MA: Harvard University Press.

Wade, M.G., Hoover, J.H., Newell, K.M., (1983). Training and trainability in motor skills performance of mentally retarded persons. In J. Hagg & P.J. Mittler (Eds.), *Advances in mental handicap research* (Vol. 2, pp. 175–201). New York: John Wiley.

Wade, M.G., Newell, K.M., & Hoover, J.H. (1982). Coincident timing behavior in young mentally handicapped workers under varying conditions of target velocity and exposure. *American Journal of Mental Deficiency*, **86**, 643–649.

Wall, A.E. (1982). Physically awkward children: A motor development perspective. In J.P. Das, R.F. Mulcahy, & A.E. Wall (Eds.), *Theory and research in learning disabilities* (pp. 253–268). New York: Plenum Press.

Wall, A.E., McClements, J., Bouffard, M., Findlay, H., & Taylor, M.J. (1985). A knowledge-based approach to motor development: Implications for the physically awkward. *Adapted Physical Activity Quarterly, 2,* 21–42.

Walton, J.N., Ellis, E., & Court, S.D.M. (1962). Clumsy children: Developmental apraxia and agnosia. *Brain, 85,* 603–615.

Weiner, B. (Ed.). (1974). *Achievement motivational attribution theory.* Morristown, NJ: General Learning Press.

Weiss, M.R. (1987). Self-esteem and achievement in children's sport and physical activity. In D. Gould & M.R. Weiss (Eds.), *Advances in pediatric sport sciences: Vol. 2. Behavioral issues* (pp. 87–119). Champaign, IL: Human Kinetics.

Wiegersma, P.H., & Velde, A., van der. (1983). Motor development of deaf children. *Journal of Child Psychology and Psychiatry, 24,* 103–111.

World Health Organization. (1980). *International classifications of impairments, disabilities and handicaps.* Geneva: Author.